BECAUSE I WAS BROKEN

Turning Weakness into Strength

By: Jacqueline Cowlin

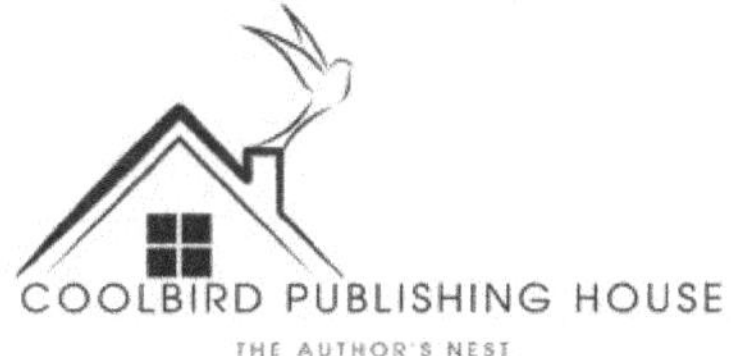

 For More information and bulk orders visit: www.jcowlinsbooks.com

ISBN 978-0-578-96166-8
Printed in the United States of America
Library of Congress Cataloging -in- Publication Data

Cover Design by: Jakeyla Cowlin
Owner of Create with Key
www.createwithkey.com

Published by: CoolBird Publishing House
www.coolbirdstudios.com

This book is dedicated to:

My children, Jakeyla and James, my grandson,
Kyler and my loving sister, Inger.

Acknowledgments

I would like to thank the key people who inspired me and helped me throughout my life. These people have been the backbone behind the scenes of my will to overcome all the obstacles in my life.

My mom and dad, Annie and Nolan have always been supportive and an inspiration in my life.

My brother, Robert aka Doobie has always been by my side and given me the utmost respect.

My sisters, Inger aka Popeye and Shaquanda are my best friends who have always had my best interest at heart. They have never let me down and have supported me in everything that I have done.

My children, Jakeyla and James are the blessings that have kept me going because of their continuous encouragement and inspiration. I am so proud of the adults that they have become.

Lastly, I want to acknowledge all my relatives and friends that support me faithfully.

Special Note: I love my grandson, Kyler, who captured my heart from the first time I heard his heartbeat.

BECAUSE I WAS BROKEN

Turning Weakness into Strength

By: Jacqueline Cowlin

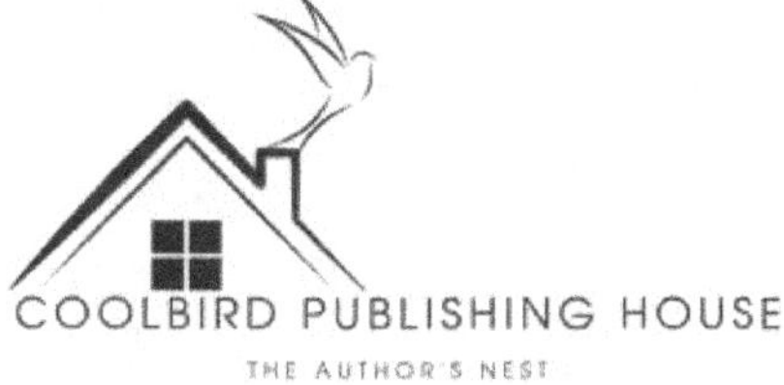

Contents

Introduction

Because I was Broken will allow you to take a journey with me as I share events that not only made me stronger, but also helped me realize just how precious life is regardless of any circumstance. I decided to write this book to give my testimony on just how blessed I am, so each page is intended to encourage you and to let you know that you are not alone. It is evident that everyone will eventually go through a situation that will help build or break you. In my case, what broke me, was also what built me. During these experiences I learned that I had to continue to be the person I am and not let anyone stop my blessings. My ultimate goal for putting pen to paper was to write a book that would inspire others because you need to know that when God has a plan for you, He'll make a way for you. The contents of this book are true and are not intended to humiliate anyone, but to explain how I became the person I am today.

-Jackie

Chapter 1

Perfectly Imperfect

Imperfect means not perfect; faulty or incomplete. All the imperfect things I have encountered has made me who I am today. When I said that you are not alone, I meant it…I've been there. Bad Marriage. Diagnosed with two diseases. Lost two friends on two different occasions who were both murdered. You see, those obstacles became the very thing that I needed to help me develop strength and courage both of which helped me become a better person. I thought that being broken was a downfall, but in actuality God used it to uplift my spirit.

My name is Jacqueline Cowlin. Most people call me Jackie. I'm a 5ft 8in tall, slender, light complexion African American woman. I'm ambitious, loyal, outgoing and as of today, I'm rocking a baldhead. The baldhead happened after I went through chemo in 2017. People always notice my eyes and I think they change color according to the season. I have been struggling with trying to gain weight. It truly is harder than everyone thinks. The stress of my past marriage and two illnesses didn't help much either.

Every day I wake up feeling blessed not because everything is perfect, but because I know that God is in control and is going to work it out for me. A woman's strength isn't just about how much she has been through in her life, it's all about how much she must handle and endure after she is broken.

I thought that having it all was the answer to building and making me a successful person. It wasn't until things started to affect my life that I realized I was broken. I was so caught up into trying to uphold an image so no one would know just how broken I was. I was strong for everyone. In my mind, I thought that I had to be strong for everyone because they relied on me. I would feel disappointed if I couldn't do for them or have what they needed even though they didn't lookout for me in the same manner.

Everyone is always telling me how strong I am, and I'm honored, but the road to being strong is definitely a struggle. The marriage was a big part of finding my strength and insight on what I needed to do and where I needed to go. In time, I learned to be patient and how a good man is supposed to treat a good woman. I've learned that when you're in a relationship that drains you, you will soon discover what it takes to build you up. I took what my ex-husband did and learned from some of his carelessness. It takes a hopeless woman to look for love within a married man. Some of these women wanted a life that he painted…a complete illusion.

As tiring as that situation was, I never let another woman take rest in my head. My family would shelter me from being hurt and try to keep me from doing things that they thought wasn't good for me. I knew they loved me, but if I allowed this to happen within my marriage, how could I be strong? I soon realized that I had to be stronger than the things I was going through.

Let me start with the first stage of being broken. I was in a relationship with a guy during high school that everyone thought was a gift to all women because he was an excellent basketball player. That same guy cheated on me with my cousin. He had me so stressed out. I was so hurt because this same cousin was one that I had confided in, and to add fuel to a burning fire…they ended up having a child together. He had people thinking that I was stalking him and evidently, they believed him. If only they knew how he was showing up at places that I was attending. I don't know why people thought that I was desperate. I guess it was easy to believe, but what they didn't know was that this handsome hometown boy was abusive.

I can remember one year my classmates and I were home for the holidays. One night we all got together and went to the club. They rode with me, but after the club they left with their boyfriend. At the time, I didn't have a boyfriend. I gave one of my friend's the keys to get her purse out of my car and she forgot to lock the door back. When I got in my car I was headed home and all of a sudden that abusive ex-boyfriend jumped out of the backseat causing me to swerve my car! This man scared the life out of me! He was yelling at me about not answering his calls and saying I had been acting funny. I told him that I was done with the relationship.

Can you believe that he had the nerve to ask me to take him home? Well, I did, and I regret it 'til this day. We talked and he tried to have sex with me. I told him that I didn't want to, but he didn't listen. I fought, but he was stronger than me. I felt like Celie on the *Color Purple*. When he was done with his business, he told me he loved me and I was sitting there thinking, "How can you love someone when you just raped me!" He told me if I tell him that I didn't love him, that he would leave me alone. I told him that I didn't love him, but the next thing I remember seeing was spots because he had slapped me so hard…I was stunned! He kept me there until I said I loved him and would come back to see him. I was with him for five hours.

Those hours were so intense and horrifying. While sitting there I remember thinking, "These people think you are a man, but you are a coward!" I finally was able to leave his house and I didn't see him anymore although he tried to connect with me. He would tell people that I was trying to "buy" him. He would tell anyone that was interested in me, that I was calling him or had been with him and it was all lies.

Years later he found out that I was getting married and showed up at my job. He threatened me and my manager had to intervene. I called my fiancé at the time, and he came to my job and waited in the parking lot. My ex never showed back up. I had gotten married, and believe it or not, my ex was in the neighborhood that I moved to… I told my husband, but he thought I was paranoid.

A guy my husband knew told him that he had seen him and picked up. The guy said that my ex was telling him that he was waiting on the opportunity to get me alone so he could get me back. My husband bought a gun and he had people looking out for him. After all that trauma, I began locking all doors and checking the backseat before getting into any car. I was terrified of relationships, but I had to be strong for me. I could not let this guy intimidate me. I was fortunate to meet my husband because he showed me so much love when we were dating. He protected and respected me. He made me feel secure and loved during the times I needed him most.

The ole' adage that says all good things will come to an end proved true with my new husband. He changed after we were married, and I ended up being in a marriage that was stressful and painful. I became numb after the cheating and lies. I could not understand how I gave this man all of me, and in return, he was so disrespectful and ungrateful. I learned that if a person is unhappy, being in a toxic relationship is not going to make it any better.

The man that I loved and wanted to live the rest of my life with was not ready to be married. I could have accepted this decision instead of being lied to. I would have done just about anything for him so that he could be happy all the while ignoring my own happiness. My faith in God was restored one Sunday after I got confirmation from hearing Reverend Cameron Thomas preach at church. It was a true God sent Word! Everything I am going through is a testimony and not a tragedy. I am still going through it, but now I'm handling it better. No matter what I'm going through, I'm always uplifted by my daughter, Jakeyla Cowlin, my parents, my sisters, Inger and Shaquanda Coleman, my brother, Robert Williams, and one of my good friend's, Stephanie Chapman!

When I look back on my life, I see pain, hurt, mistakes and heartaches. Yet, when I look in the mirror, I see strength, lessons learned and pride in myself. I continue to work on improving myself because I want to become better. Everyone sees a strong woman in me, and I'm grateful. It is hard sometimes trying to be strong when everything is coming at me. ***I found out the hard way that sometimes when people say they wish you "well" or that they are for you only means that the "well" they are wishing you turns into a dam, and that they are not really for you, but secretly against you.***

There was once a time in my life when I needed approval from people until I realized that God is the only one that has a plan for me, and His approval is the only one that I need. I had a very close friend of mine to pass. And during that time, I didn't have faith in anything especially after being diagnosed with my illness. Eventually, I began to regain my faith. I did not go to church as much as some people, but that didn't mean my faith was any less.

Regrettably, others did not think that my faith in God was as strong as theirs because of my lack of attendance in church. I knew my faith was just as strong because of all the things that God was doing and still is doing for me. God has spared my life in so many incidents because He has a plan for me. I know that I am doing something right because He has kept me here. I also realize that the topic of church is a touchy subject, and a lot of people love their church and their pastors. Trust me, I don't blame them for being loyal to a Pastor who is faithful and loyal to God.

When I would go to church, I was sometimes approached by members saying, "It's good to see you, but don't make this your last time coming." I didn't know how to take that. I thought about it, and I concluded that it was offensive and then I grew angry. This particular member would continue to say those kinds of things to me. Each time I felt hurt, but I still respected her.

One day I was fed up. I said, "Ma'am, I might not be at church every Sunday like you, because I work on

Sunday's, and I have a child to feed. I do have faith and I refuse to let you steal my joy and faith in God." Since then, she has never said that to me again. How do people expect someone to come to church with those kinds of remarks? Eventually, I stopped going and started looking for another church, even though I loved my Pastor.

Our Pastor retired and then we had another Pastor. A lot of people talked about how good he could preach. I went to hear him a few times and he was good with words. After being diagnosed with cancer, my stepsister came to me about a benefit program. The guy that was going to organize it asked me about my church helping to participate. I told him that truthfully, I was considered an inactive member.

I called and talked to the Pastor that was there and I asked him about participating, but he was negative about the organization that was doing the benefit program. The organization was the Mason's. This Pastor did not want to get involved because he said that it was a cult and I told him that wasn't true. I was disappointed because I did not expect this.

I called the guy who wanted to organize the benefit program and told him what I was told, and he was furious. He told me not to worry and that he has it covered. Well, he did organize it and it was nice. Some of my classmates and friends that I hadn't seen in a while attended. A few members of the church showed up too.

The things about the church that I am speaking of has changed. I once felt that the love and the Word was touching and fit, but the last straw that really tore my soul was when I came to church after I was better with my treatments. The Pastor was preaching and the words that came out of his mouth were, "You say you have cancer, but your hair is growing back!" He turns to look at me and our eyes met. He lost his concentration and changed the ending. Everyone was yelling amen until he said this because everyone knew that the cancer person with no hair was me.

The devil was on me because I wanted to run up there and hit him in his freaking throat. How dare you come for me after all the things that I have endured. I am still upset about my hair. I felt like he was implying that I was lying about having Cancer. Every time I see him or his sermons on Facebook, that moment replays in my head. I don't know how I am supposed to get over this. I have not let this alter my faith, but I thought the man of God was supposed to uplift the faith of the church. This is the church that I joined when I was a little girl. ***I am still seeking a church that treats me***

as a member whether I go every day or once a month. I am not a fan of those who base their sermons on the ones that come to church less than the other members.

When a person joins or comes to church, their sins should not be pointed out to the congregation. That person needs a prayer to help them to be better. I know talking about the church is a touchy subject, but it must be said. I was at church one time and this Pastor was supposedly prophesizing about a marriage. I was embarrassed for the couple. I would have thought that God would have told him to speak to the couple and not discuss it in front of the congregation. I learned that we must please God and not worry about the judgement of others. I used to wonder why people were always being blessed even when they would manipulate and treat others wrong.

I thought that when you do good, then good things would come to me. I realized that good things do come to me because I am still blessed. The little blessings are the ones that are the most powerful. Just knowing that I woke up the next morning. I am grateful to see another birthday, to enjoy my family and friends, and to see the day that I became a grandmother. I never thought that my life had any meaning until I realized the meaning of having life. It took me to almost lose my life in order to appreciate living. I was struggling with myself to be better than I was at the time.

I never thought that being imperfect would be the key to being strong and encouraging. I would think that everything in life must be perfect for life to be great. I found that this is not true. Things must happen imperfectly for a person to appreciate their life. Sometimes, God will make you wait on purpose so that you know it was His favor. See, I've been let down by people that I thought would be by my side, but I never let up. I have been set up to be lied on, cheated on and to fail, but it did not set me back. When the devil wanted me to give in, I did not give in…Instead, I raised up.

When people turned their back and quit on me, I bounced back stronger. You see, I did not quit on the one person that I could count on, me. Because of my faith and the plan that God has for me I survived things that should have killed me. I had to realize that everything that you go through whether good or bad, will either make or break you. It is the strength in the person that overcome the things that life presents.

I thought about writing a book but didn't know whether I should do it or not. One day as fate would have it, a publisher named Taminko Kelley reached out to me through messenger on Facebook. She said, "Jackie I have a vision of you writing a book." I was like wow! I have been battling with the thought of trying to write a book and I think this is my confirmation! Nothing but God! Then she told me that she needed eight chapters.

I was already journaling, so I had already started on my book without even knowing it. I tried to come up with eight chapters, but I only had seven. I thought to myself that I just couldn't come up with the last chapter. Then, my sister passed and there was my eighth chapter. The eighth chapter that Taminko Kelley envisioned. The eighth chapter was hard to write. I did not realize that I was actually writing this chapter all alone.

When I was in the hospital with my sister, I would write details about how I felt and what she was experiencing during her ordeal with Breast Cancer. I had to write about it because I did not want her to know that I was worried. I did not want her to know that I was scared, I could not tell my family about my thoughts or concerns because they were already scared, confused and angry…and so was I.

I had a bad feeling that I just could not shake. I kept thinking, "Why am I feeling this way? She will be alright."

Even though I knew she would be alright, I was not at peace with her leaving me. I needed my sister to laugh and joke with.

I was caught off-guard with these two diseases which made me stronger. I was scared, but ready to take on the fight. My children were my greatest supporters. They kept me encouraged and made sure that I was always taken care of. I don't think my fight would have been that powerful if it weren't for my children. I wanted to raise them. I wanted to instill my moral and values into them. God helped me to make that possible. In me I see POWER. Picture Of a Woman Everyone Respects.

I had this person who wanted to be in my life at a time when I would not let him. He was trying to be there when my marriage was going wrong, when I was sick, when I was talked about, and when I almost lost everything, he is a good man. No! a GREAT man. I finally let my guard down because of the hurt and pain to let him in my life. It has been a true blessing because he has been there for me ever since. I just want everyone to know who he is. He is GOD. Thank you, God!

Chapter 2

The Marriage

Facebook Post | May 2011

What's on my mind? Sick and tired of being labeled a mad, angry or bitter BLACK woman! Excuse me if I am mad, angry, or bitter because I am the ONLY parent that is putting OUR child through school but not the ONLY parent that is getting recognition! I can care less about what he does as a man, but as a father, I do get bitter when I am the only parent in three years that sacrifice to make sure she has what is needed but he wants to brag!

People often get the anger of what women have towards their baby daddy's and misconstrue about what they don't do as a father with the woman being angry and bitter because of who the man is with. Not all of us are that woman. We work jobs we hate; we don't eat or sleep so our children can, we put our children needs before our own. We don't regret it; just reassure our children of our strength.

I have been through so much these past 6 months. Lied to, lied on, trusting people that I thought had my well-being at heart but selfishly had their own interests. I have always given unconditionally to everyone in my life. I have had my bank account compromised by a fraudulent company that took all my money! Then, my income stopped, I'm going through health issues, been lied on and I'm travelling back and forth taking care of my dad and much more. Worst of all, I'm slowly losing my faith in yes, God...-

Every girl wants to find the man of her dreams. I married the man that I thought was the love of my life. I wanted to have a child by this man. I met him through my best friend. She thought we would make a great couple because we both were in bad relationships. I never thought that I would ever fall in love with anyone else. I kept out of committed relationships for a while.

The relationship that I was involved in before I got married was horrible. Lamar came along at a time in my life when things were bad. He was so supportive and knew all the right things and words to say. I was taken by his suave attributes. When we went out on our first date, I came to pick him up. I went to his mother's house. He wasn't ready so I had to wait in the basement which was like a den. His mother's home was very nice.

While I was in the basement watching television, this tall medium build, pretty woman comes downstairs. She looks as though she has been running or exercising. I speak to her, and she speaks back dryly. I said, "My name is Jackie, I'm a friend of Lamar's. Do you run or something because you look good?" With a deep and strong voice, she said, "I am Sherry, Lamar's mother…I walk every day." I said, "Well, you look good!" We started talking about so many things and discovered that she knew my mom and grandmother.

Her mother and my grandmother were friends. Lamar came downstairs and peaked in the room and then went back upstairs. Later there was a knock at the front door. Mrs. Sherry excused herself and went to answer it. Soon after, Lamar came downstairs to tell me that we can't go out because his baby mother has dropped his son off. In my mind, I was thinking, "Boy I did not come all this way to hang out with your fine tail and now your baby mama thinks she is going to mess this up!" So, I calmly said, "Why he can't go with us?" He looked surprised and said, "Are you sure?" I said "Yes, we are going out to eat and to the movies, right?" He said, "Yes!" He kissed me and went upstairs to get his son ready.

We left and I enjoyed myself. His son, Ladarius was taken by me; He held my hand and sat by me. He was handsome and flirts like his dad. Ladarius was sleep when we got back to Lamar's mom house. Lamar gave me a kiss and said, "Thank you." I said, "For what?" He said, "For accepting my son." I said, "Well, if we are going to be in a relationship, then your kids are a part of that so I'm cool." He kisses me again. I could have melted. I drove home thinking about him and this situation. I knew I was going to have to handle this baby mama if I was going to continue with him…And I was ready. As time went by, his baby mother realized that I wasn't going anywhere, and eventually we got along fine.

We got married on January 9, 1993. I found out that I was three months pregnant. He seemed incredibly happy about the pregnancy. He wanted a girl who would look just like him. He started out giving me a lifestyle that spoiled me during my pregnancy. We had our daughter on July 17,1993. She was beautiful! She was what made my life worth living. My daughter and stepson have been the most amazing thing that came out of my broken marriage. They made me keep going no matter what.

He seemed very happy about our little family. He loved his daughter. She looked just like him with my skin complexion. That made his day! He treated me like a queen. My daughter and her father have so many ways alike. I sometimes felt like I was an outsider. She was getting her hair and nails done at four years old. He spoiled her. I was the mean parent who did the discipline. But I was respected. He would be scared to discipline her. I would ask him what could she do besides get mad? She's two! She doesn't pay bills and can't beat anything. I would tell him not to make her helpless and that I need for her to be strong! I made sure she earned everything she received. She would learn to appreciate everything that she earned and received.

I did run into a few situations with other women. I would get my respect by getting ahead of the situation. They called me crazy, but I called it getting respect. No woman has ever replaced what we had; they just filled a space. We would hang out with his friends and partners a lot. I had the respect of them all. They knew what I was like. We went out to eat with his little friend, Brook. At the time, Lamar was broke so I was the one paying for the food.

The waitress was attentive to Lamar. Pouring him refills, bringing extra rolls and meanwhile I'm sipping on ice cubes. So, I tell him that he needs to handle her before I go off, but I didn't. I exchanged our glasses and told Brook to watch this. She ran over to refill my glass that I put in front of him. He looked at me and said, "WHAT? She did not give me service; she gave you service." She brought the check and put the check in front of him. I took the check and put the money on the table to pay for the check. Lamar said, "Jazzy, are you going to tip her?" I said, "Oh yeah...Next time know who is paying the check, while you are running over here filling up his glass, he's broke! Wait on his tip!" I walked toward the door. She just stood there. Lamar said to me, "Jazzy, she's just doing her job."

My marriage was not the best by far. We went through things like others but ours was showcased because of who we were. Lamar promised me the world. He promised me that he would never hurt me or betray me for anyone. Those promises became empty after three years. No matter what- I stayed loyal, honest and by his side through it all. I get asked why? He was my husband. I kept remembering the things he did for me. He stayed by my side through troubling times, and he protected me. He reassured me that I was safe with him. You know… that type of man.

He made me feel like we were equal on everything. I fell in love with this man. I thought I was his rib but found out he had a slab. I made jokes out of some of the situations to keep from crying. If I cried, it was bad. My family loved him despite his cheating. They knew about his cheating but didn't say a word. I wish they would have, maybe things would've been different.

Lamar started out spoiling me with everything that I wanted. I would shop every Friday with no limit. I loved every minute of it. When we got married, he became different. But first, let me say this, when you get married and you support your vows, you stick to your vows. You are not stupid or whatever these people call you. You are just doing what you stated in front of God. It's the one who doesn't abide by the vows that should be wearing the black eye. But no! Everyone puts the black eye on the innocent one.

I had a husband that thought that I had to be with him and there for him. You know loyalty! I was. He became complacent with me, and I was complacent with him too. I was the "wifey". I was the one who kept him from going down while breaking into pieces. Did he see the pieces? No. I had to be the strong one and the one who kept it together, while falling into pieces. As long as, I was beautiful, loyal and intelligent, he remained happy. I was around powerful people who respected me and trusted me. I was the strongest woman they knew.

Nobody ever knew how broken I was. They knew of the illness as being a weakness; it was also my strength, and it will continue to be. Everything about me was real. Being real became my brand. Although my brand was well represented, the pieces of my life, was breaking. I was at that moment where I started realizing that my marriage was over. I couldn't do it anymore. I was tired, scared and fed up.

These things make a woman dangerous. I was tired of all the lies and cheating. The cheating had become normal in my marriage. It was turning me bitter and dangerous. I couldn't be controlled anymore.

My marriage and life were more complicated than people lied about. Everyone always had things to report about my marriage. It wasn't the best marriage, but I obtained wonderful children who I love dearly. Lamar, my ex-husband was cheating. He cheated when we were dating. It's true that marriage does not make anything better, it infact made things worse. I was consumed with him. My life was about him at first. He took care of me, but his appetite for women was overwhelming.

He preyed on the insecure women and made them feel beautiful. He would discuss my passions for purses, shoes and lifestyle. They wanted what I had but wasn't aware of the consequences that were behind the things I was accustomed to at that time. I liked that we were a team. We were opposites but it worked. Lamar and I worked. At times I had to break him down about who is really the powerful one between the two of us. He would get so excited about the reputation. That's just what it was...a reputation.

My life wasn't a fairy tale, but it was a mystery with manipulation, lies and deceit. I encountered people who would scare and intimidate the average person. I'm the wild card. The one everyone least expect. I was considered as the nice person. I can be nice. People really had the relationship twisted.

It was assumed that because he was handsome and charming, which the women were taken by him, that I was obsessed with him. It's funny because I had lots of opportunities to be unfaithful, but my loyalty was stronger to a weak man. I called him weak because if he couldn't be faithful or loyal then all he had to do was say it. They thought that I couldn't do anything without him, but it was him that couldn't do without me. He needed me.

At first, he thought that I couldn't do anything without him or that I would need him. We broke up and then everything was revealed. I have come across a few women that I had to check only because of trying to disrespect me! Everyone sees me as little quiet Jackie. I am, but don't push me. I had to display a character that they were not familiar with. I would tell them that he was just out for fun. He's not going anywhere until I say it's over. And that's what happened.

When I got sick and tired, I was done with that situation. I kept breaking and then trying to put the pieces back together and would break again. I would pray and ask God for guidance or a sign to show me where I needed to be…Can I do this alone? He would show me in my dreams about another woman. The women would still be surfacing and I knew that I was unhappy. I would ignore the signs that I had asked for and things got deeper and deeper. I wasn't ready to give up on this marriage or the man because I didn't want to be alone or start over.

He made me think that nobody would want me, and that he was the best person for me. He would say he's handling some business and would be late coming home. This wasn't unusual because of his business. I always said that I understood but didn't believe him. There were times it wouldn't make since and I would question him about the lie I caught him in. I would even tell him that he better gets his chick on lock down because her name keeps buzzing. He always laughed.

When my daughter was born, I became stronger and determined to make sure she wasn't exposed to the things her dad did. The first time Lamar cheated on me; I was hurt. He was out for a long period. Nobody knew it mainly because I kept my marriage business in my home. I would lay next to him thinking of ways to kill him. The more I thought about the cheating, the angrier I got. I thought about putting the gun to his head and unloading it. I decided to get out of bed with him before I killed him. So, I got up and went to sleep with my daughter. I couldn't forgive or forget. He never knew my intentions. He knew I was dangerous, but he didn't know how much. I became distant and cautious. I could not trust him anymore. I couldn't stand the sight of him. I began to see him for what he was- selfish and self-centered.

He wasn't the person that I fell in love with anymore. Lamar didn't have respect for the marriage or my health. As the marriage went downhill, I began to prepare to get out of this situation. He didn't realize that he was losing me. He just saw it as an opportunity to be with other women. I didn't care anymore because my heart was cold and damaged. He was supportive for the wrong reasons.

He came home one day and was so inquisitive about my health, my doctor appointment and my symptoms. I was so excited! He was trying to be involved. Nope! His Aunt Norma came home and was asking him questions about my health and was trying to see if he was knowledgeable about

Lupus. He wasn't. He told me that she told him that he needed to know all about my health issues the next time she comes home because my situation was serious. I was sitting there with my mouth wide open. He wasn't concerned because he cared but because he wanted to impress his aunt.

When my best friend was killed, I knew in my gut who the killer was. This was one of the most damaging days of my life. My faith in God was questioned. I couldn't believe this happened to me. She was such an amazing individual. My heart was torn. I couldn't breathe. Lamar was there to help me breathe. He helped me to see that she was in a better place. He kept me safe. He reassured me that it was going to be alright. He stayed for the tears, the pain and the heartbreak. He was my protector. For me, this was the beginning of a bond. We began to trust each other. We both had things in our life that were similar. I was taken by the way Lamar spoiled me.

I think that I was the only woman who did not bow down to him. He likes to be in control and wanted the upper hand, but I wasn't the one to fold. I was probably the first to tell him, no. I basically had attention from men just as he did with women. He didn't know how to handle someone who was not insecure. Later I figured out that he preyed on insecure women. The women who were infatuated with him, gave him power.

During our marriage, he was always cheating. I think he was amazed by his cousin, Disco. Disco was a habitual cheater. He was awe-struck by me, and he had the utmost respect for me. Everyone who knew us, knew this. Some of our acquaintances thought we were fooling around. I remember the first time we talked. He had this very deep voice and it was sexy.

I loved talking to him. He was funny and a joy to be around. Lamar had gone to visit him so they could do some work together. I didn't want Lamar to go because I was six months pregnant. But we needed the money, so I went along with the idea. During this time, I had not met Disco yet and only held conversations with him over the phone.

There were no cellphones at the time, so I would call to the location they were supposed to be at to talk to Lamar, and he was never available! I was getting upset each time I called. I did get a chance to talk to his cousin Disco and I told him to tell Lamar to call me or else I'm coming up there with a one-way ticket for him and a round trip ticket for me! I told him to tell Lamar that when I come, he needs to be ready to leave and that I was not playing because he has a wife and a child on the way! Disco said that he would deliver the message. Lamar finally called me but was upset at the threat I made. I didn't care that he was mad. I just needed him to do what I said. I reiterated what I said to Disco, and he knew I meant every word.

One Sunday evening a big Mercedes pulled up in the yard. I hear this voice and I know it's Disco's voice, but when he got out the car, he was about 5'8" and was small. I was disappointed because his voice was deep and sexy. I thought he would be 6 feet tall and muscular. He saw me and said, "Dang Lamar! Your wife is beautiful! I see why you had to get back." Disco came over and hugged me. He said to Lamar, "Boy! You better be glad you met her first because I would take her from you." I thought to myself, "Oh no! you are not my type. I would not have given you a second look."

From that point on, Disco and I became the best of friends. People thought that we had something going on. But my husband didn't think that about me. He knew I was loyal. Disco just had respect for me. He would keep in touch with me and made sure that I was taken care of you know, the things that my husband should have done. My husband worked hard at being with the ladies. If he had of worked that hard in getting and saving money, he could have been in a good place by now. I was the one who took care of having fall back money.

He always made the statement that it wasn't me that ruined our marriage and that it was him and blamed it on being young. It was always an excuse as to why he had not grown into a responsible man. I wanted to just be happy and have that perfect marriage with the husband, wife, and child.

Every little girl always dreams of their prince charming, and I thought Lamar was my prince charming. We started out being best friends. We would talk for hours and see each other every weekend. Then we got married and things changed. I found out I was pregnant, and I was scared. Although I was grown and married, I didn't know how to tell my mom. When I did tell her, she was excited, and my grandmother said I was almost too old.

The marriage took me to points in my life that I am not proud of. But at the same time, it helped me to develop into a powerful person mentally. I endured a lot of unhappiness, but I was so determined to have a marriage even if I wasn't happy. My husband would stay out for days as though he did not have a family. I was only necessary when he wanted to impress important people who respected me. The marriage became more of a business. I looked away at the cheating for a long time until I got tired. I was loyal to someone who stressed that people weren't loyal, but he was not loyal to the woman who held his back. The woman who kept him out of the grave.

People always seem to judge the one that is cheated on for being weak or stupid. Love…That four letter word is more powerful than anyone can imagine.

The Infidelities

Part of my breakdown was due to the disrespect along with the cheating. It took away parts of my heart that made it almost impossible to be able to completely love a man. The infidelities had hit my life very hard, and I was so caught off guard. I stayed in my marriage for the sake of my children and eventually realized that they were hurting just as much.

At this point, I knew it was time for me to let this situation go…It had to end. The first time I found out Lamar was cheating; it tore me to pieces, and I was devastated. I kept it to myself but unfortunately everyone knew about him cheating. I was ashamed that I could not fulfill my wifely duties. After being diagnosed with Lupus, I could not stand for Lamar to touch me. Whenever he would come home, I would lie still just so he wouldn't touch me or wouldn't want to have sex. I couldn't stand for him to breathe on me. At one point, I did not care that he was seeing another woman just so he wouldn't bother me.

I could not tolerate the pain of the body contact; I could not satisfy my husband sexually because of the pain. I would later ignore the cheating because I was feeling guilty about not fulfilling my wifely duties. He had no respect for me. I did not fault the woman because it was Lamar who I was married to; He took the vows. He cared more about being in the streets and honestly, I never tried to keep him from those streets.

The first time I found out he cheated on me was after we were married, and I was devastated. After I gave birth to my daughter, I was released to go and he wasn't there to pick me up. It was humiliating because I had to find someone to pick me up from the hospital. Yes, it was tragic. When he finally came home, he had red hickey marks all over his neck. Can you believe that he had the nerve to try and convince me that I was the one who did it? Then, everything hit me. "This is what you have been doing all along? You got to go, and you got to get out now! I want a divorce!" I screamed. He pleaded with me that he didn't want a divorce and left long enough for me to cool down, but I didn't cool down. I was hurt and I was angry! He was gone for months and yes, he was with her. He would send messages to me, and I ignored them. I just couldn't understand why he would jeopardize his family. I was a loyal dedicated woman. He finally came to see his child and he wanted to come back, but I couldn't let him.

I guess the woman who he was with realized that he wanted to come back, so she called me. Ummm…Wow! She told me that he said he had asked for a divorce and wanted to marry her. I said, "No! I was the one who wanted the divorce, but if that's what he wants, then it's fine with me." The divorce never happened. The woman was older than both of us with kids. It's always fun and exciting when a person is out being deceitful until they are forced to be with the person.

It was one thing to be disrespectful, but to be seen with her around my hometown. Everyone kept it from me because I was dealing with Lupus and stayed sick. I understood that they didn't want me to be upset, but I think I needed to know because I knew how to handle the situation.

I did tell him to get out, but I was hurt because I was still in love with him, and I didn't want to lose him. My head knew he wasn't any good for me, but my heart was in love. I had people to tell me what they would and would not do or put up with.

It is always easy for a person to tell you their thoughts especially if they have never been in your shoes. Truth be told, some of the advice that was given needed to be taken by the person that was giving it. I thought that I wanted this man. I needed this marriage and I needed for this man to love me as I loved him.

Women who date married men are under the impression that he loves them and will leave their wife. In my case, my husband used the excuse that she is sick, and I just can't leave her right now. He even said he wasn't married, or that I was just a baby mama. They are gullible to believe that they will leave their wives and not being realistic. I think it's called karma- if he did it to me, he will do the same thing to them.

I never fought for my husband to be home with me if he cheated. I just let him go be with whomever he was cheating with. If he was working that hard to cheat with her then just go. Of course, after he was there for a couple of weeks, the cheating wasn't that special anymore. I know that I shouldn't have let it go on for as long as I did, but it is what it is. I felt like no other man would want a woman that was sick. So, I stayed with a man that did what I feared and that was to be cheated on. He didn't want me- I was in a marriage by myself. I would find out that he was cheating and warned him that I knew.

This first chick, Cent, would do things to let me know he was with her. He would tell lies and wanted me to think that it was in my mind. It was bad enough that he was cheating, but he started having her to pick him up in my hometown. Later I found out that he was also messing with one of my cousins who was friends with Cent. Then he dumped her and started back dating Cent...It be your own folks.

This was not the only cousin that he has dealt with. Yes, he was trifling, and they were too. When Cent felt like she was being replaced, she contacted me to inform me of her replacement. At first, I thought this chick was crazy. I didn't care about who he was with because he was out of my place. But she was right, he did have another chick.

Lamar preyed on insecure women who was impressed by his fantasy life...the one he created to tell them. The insecure women were the ones he could control and manipulate. He loved the ones who were amazed with him telling them he was from Chicago. In actuality he was born and raised from a town called Childersburg, Alabama. The women loved his looks. At first, I was taken by his looks too, but I knew the accent and where he was from was not real.

Cent had informed me of the other woman who had taken her place. Yes, the girlfriend called the wife to tell of her replacement. This chick did not know he was married. She was younger. One day I got a note saying call a certain number. I called and it's this chick named Dawn.

Dawn was a simple chick. I felt sorry for her because I knew that Lamar had manipulated her. I knew she was taken by his looks and lies. Lamar could tell these women things to make them think they were a supermodel. I'm not saying she was unattractive, but I became amazed by the women he was with but after a while it didn't surprise me.

When I made the phone call, I was very polite with her because it was not her fault. She was very apologetic. I explained to her the situation. Every woman thought that I was telling them something for them to let go. It was never like that. Contrary to popular belief, I let him go to be with these women. I wasn't insecure. I was confident in myself. I did not stand in his way. I did not need the drama. As I sit back and think about how easy it was for me to let him go, maybe I didn't love him as much as I thought. I guess I could say that I loved him enough to let him be happy, even if it meant that he wasn't going to be with me.

That relationship went on for longer than it should have lasted. I got a phone call from one of my best friends named Tip. She told me that she needed to tell me something…I said, "Okay." She told me that while she was at the Beauty Shop, she heard Lamar's aunts having a conversation. She said they were talking about how his mom was upset with him because he had brought a baby to her house and said it was his. They said that she was upset and told him to take that baby back to the mama because she was not impressed. She said that his mom said Jackie is a good woman and wife and you are not going to disrespect her because I love her. She also said his mom told him to take that baby back and get out. They said she was mad. Tip said she also heard them say how good you were to him. I told Tip thank you for telling me and after all she had said, my heart could have burst.

I had so many emotions going through my head. Tip told me that I could tell him that she was the one who told me what was said. I told her okay…thanks and I'll let her know what happens. I got off the phone and called him. He answered and I said, "Hey Baby! What are you doing?" He said that he was working. I said, I miss you. What time are you coming home? I have something planned for you. He said "really?" I said, "yes." He told me that he should be home in a couple of hours. I said just call me when you reach Sylacauga, Alabama. He said, bet! I said to myself, that's just enough time to go to Walmart to get a new lock for my doors.

I went and got new locks and changed them, packed his clothes and waited on his call. Lamar finally called to say that he was in Sylacauga, so I went and sat by the door. He pulled up and I opened the door. He walked in and gave me a hug and kiss. He saw that I had on a jogging suit with sneakers. I said have a seat and then I began telling him what was said.

He was about to lie, but I told him who had told me. He dropped his head and said yes, it's true but I didn't know how to tell you. I said you didn't know how to tell me, but you knew how to bring her around your mother? He told me

Jay we need to talk. I told him we needed to talk when he knew that chick was pregnant. I told him that he was so disrespectful, that his clothes were packed, and that he must go! I told Lamar that this has gotten to be old and don't call me. He said, "But Jay." I interrupted him and said there is nothing you can say or do. Just go! He left and I sat there despising him. I did not cry but I wanted to punch him. I called to have my number changed. I didn't talk to Lamar for 6 months. He called family and friends telling lies. He called my grandmother and told her that I had left home saying that I was coming down to her house, but he hasn't heard from me since.

My grandmother called me all upset and I had to tell her what happened and that he was lying. I would never tell my family what was going on in my household although I had people in the family that told lies about what was going on in my house. Those are the same people who have a walk-in closet of things going on but worried about mine. I made sure that Lamar did what he was supposed to do for this little girl because it wasn't her fault that he and her mom were irresponsible.

Time did pass and our kids were now old enough for me to take them to Disney World in July. He made the arrangements for transportation, and this is also how I found out about chick number three. She was the last chick that I was going to deal with. This third chick was named Lacey and she was a nurse. Lacey had rented a car for me to go to Disney. I looked in the glove compartment and there was her information. Her name, address and phone number. I wrote it down to keep just in case I needed it for later.

Three months later, Lamar called to see if I needed anything before he came home. I said no. After he hung up, I got a phone call from a private number. I answered it and there is music in the background but no one's saying anything. When he got home, I told him to tell his girlfriend to stop calling me when you leave. He said I didn't have a girlfriend and I told him that I am warning you because the next time I'm going to call her. He laughed and I told him that I was dead serious. Of course, he swears it's nobody. I already knew the chick's name, address and phone number, but it wasn't the time to confront him. It was my ace in the hole.

One day in the summer, Lamar called to see if he could take me out of town for the weekend. I told him yes because I like to ride. We would go out of town which wasn't unusual. We left Jakeyla with my mom. He had already told my mom to call his phone if anything happened because he was taking me to get some rest. We had a good weekend, until I got a call on my cell. It wasn't unblocked or private. I called out the number and I noticed that Lamar was nervous. So, I answered just because he seemed nervous. I said, “Hello” and she said, “Hello, Jackie this is Lacey.” I said to myself this is a woman-to-woman phone call, but it better be the right kind of woman calling. She began telling me that her and Lamar has had a thing going on for about six months and that he said that he was going to leave me. I said, "Oh! He did?" I pulled back to hit him, but I didn't. Lamar did jump. She said, “He took me to get an abortion Friday. He took me to the clinic and dropped me off and then came back to pick me up. He took me home and I haven't heard from him.”

I giggled a little, because I was never going to give another woman the satisfaction of thinking she was getting to me. I’ll mess with her head first. I said to her, “So why are you calling me?” She sounded confused. She said, "I was just letting you know that he was cheating on you." I said to her, now you want to tell me he's cheating on me because when I called you a few months ago to ask were you guys involved you told me no. That was your opportunity then but now you call me after you got rid of the problem. I'm not going anywhere, and he isn't either. See, you got rid of the problem so there is no need for us to address this matter. I hung up and yes, I went upside his head. I told him you got to be the dumbest want to be player in the world. You are out here laying down with these different women with no protection, and you wonder why I won't let you touch me. So here I go again... I was so tired of Lamar.

Lamar was staying with her and as usual it wasn't what he thought. But that wasn't my business. He would be around my house lurking. I would catch him near the house. He called me one time and told me that he could have done something to me, but our child was with me. Really? I told Lamar to give those threats to the others who believed him because I am not the one honey. I never felt insecure to let you scare me, remember I have been with you to know what's real and what's not. I cannot be intimidated. Besides, if it's God's will for me to die by your hands, so let it be done. I know how you got that reputation, but remember, I am not afraid to pull the trigger with a smile.

He had a homeboy named Short and he hooked up with his cousin. I didn't like Short anyway. Her name was Tisha. Lamar also had an aunt named Tisha. I found her out by the house phone. Lamar was such a dummy when it came to cheating. Even when I warned him about knowing what he was doing. I thought that I had used the phone last, so I redialed the last number. The chick said, "Hello." I said, "Hello, who is this?" She said, "This is Tisha." I said, "Lamar's aunt?" I asked because it didn't sound like his aunt. She replied while laughing, "No, it's his girl…Who is this?" I said, "This is his wife!" She said, "He never said he had a wife!" I said, "He never said he had a girlfriend either but apparently, he got one of them too. But he does have a wife and a child…don't worry it will be handled." I hung up and put her number in my cellphone. I never said anything about the conversation, but I knew he wasn't going to say anything to me.

Well, a couple of weeks later, we were hanging out. We went to get pedicures. My grandmother was watching our daughter. They were finished with me so Lamar's phone rung. He told me to see who it was. I see the number and it's Tish. I say it's a 313-area code. He said, "Answer it. It's probably Lil Earn." I knew it wasn't Earnie because I had already called this chick and saved the number in my phone, but I was anxious to answer. I said, "Hello." She said, "Is Lamar around." I said, "He's busy." She said, "Will you have him to call Tish back?" I said, "Sure!" When I hung up the phone, he asked who it was. I told him that I would tell him later. The little Chinese man told Lamar, you in trouble. When we get in the car, I told him that it was Tish that called. He said, “Oh, Auntie?” I said, “Heck no, your girlfriend.” He said, “You call her...” Of course, he thought I didn’t know her number. I told him to call her and see what she wants. He said you call her of course thinking that I didn't know the number. I looked up the number in my phone that I had saved and called. She answered and I told her that I'm Lamar's wife the one you talked to weeks ago and the one who answered his phone an hour ago. She told me that he still said he wasn’t married. I told her he's a lie and that he also says he doesn’t have a girlfriend, but here you are! She asked where he was and if she could talk to him. I said he's right here driving, and then I gave him my phone. He said, “Hello?” and then she started asking him questions.

Meanwhile, he is answering with one word. I said if she is asking you, are you married, you need to be making complete sentences. Your answer should be no, I'm not married or yes, I'm married. Lamar started yelling at me, so I snatched my phone from him and hit him upside the head and broke my phone while telling him that he doesn't talk to me stupid in front of nobody! When we arrived at his mom’s house we looked like that scene with Ike and Tina Turner fighting in the back of the limousine. He told his mama about me hitting him, but I told her everything. Then she asked me how much did my phone cost. I told her how much and she told me that she would give me the money to buy a new one. I looked at him like I'm going to get you when we get home.

Yes, I was the abusive spouse. I did all the hitting and he laughed which made me even angrier! That's one thing about him…he has never put his hands on me. Well, he pushed me down in the bathroom one time when I came home from the club with friends. I didn't expect him to be home. When I got home there wasn't any lights on, so I said he hasn't gotten home yet. I go into the house and there he was sitting there with the lights off. I turn the lights on, and he asked me where I have been. He scared me because

I didn't think he was there, so I jumped. As I'm walking down the hall, he is following me asking me questions and I am answering the questions while trying to get a shower. He said why are you taking a shower? I said, I have been in a club, and I smell like smoke. He said yeah right, then he picks my clothes up and smells them. I said, "Boy what is the matter with you?" He pushed me back and I fell and hit my head on the tub. When I came up, I grabbed the AK47 that we kept in the bathroom. We had guns in every room of the house. I pointed it at him and told him that

I was not going to be with someone who hits on women because I grew up watching my mom and aunt running from a man who was beating on them. I told him I will never be with a man that hits me. But if you ever, put your hands on me, I promise I will bring your family, friends and girlfriends all together to say their goodbyes. He's yelling, “Jay, do you realize what you have in your hands?” as he is backing up. I told him yes, I know it will blow a hole in you and that's exactly what I want it to do. He left out of the bathroom. I was upset. I went to take a shower to calm myself down because I was mad.

After I got out of the shower, I went to bed, and he slept on the sofa that night. The next day, I got up and got ready for work and we didn’t talk to each other. He apologized when he picked me up from work. When I got home, he had cooked and ran me some bath water. We discussed what happened and made up. He promised that he would never put his hands on me, and I promised that if he didn't put his hands on me, his family, friends and girlfriends wouldn't get together. He laughed but I was dead serious. After that happened, he never did it again because if he had I promise on everything I love he would be covered in dirt.

The Divorce

The true reason why we were separated was so different from the rumors. It was told that he left me for another woman. As a matter fact, for the woman he is with now. She probably thought that too. People gave him so much power and credit for being the one to control the marriage. It was not like that. I guess because I was not sleeping around and it wasn't any juicy gossip, he had to be the one to leave. I had come home from the hospital. I was in there for weeks at a time. But this time, I had done some soul searching.

I knew that I was done with the marriage for good. I could not tolerate it any longer and I was going to discuss this with Lamar when I got home. I was so sick of the arguing that I told him to go ahead and go where you are trying to go because I don't have time for this mess you are doing. He quickly agreed to leave. He told me that he was going to his moms for a little while. I knew that was a lie. He left and I felt relieved. Although I knew he was going to be with someone else.

I did not care anymore, but he was calling every night to tell us good night and that he misses us. I just prayed for God to show me where I needed to be. I wanted him to show me if this man was for me. Lamar's mother called the house looking for him. I told her that he wasn't there and that he said he was staying with her. She was upset and told me that he was lying (*which I knew*) and that he could not live with her anymore. I told her that he has been gone for two weeks. She told me to tell him to call her if I speak to him and I said that I would. I can remember thinking to myself thank you God, I will not overlook your signs anymore.

Lamar called the house just like he did every night and I told him of the conversation that his mom and I had. He got quiet and then said we need to talk. I told him that we should have had this talk the day he left. I told him that it was somewhere else that he wanted to be and that he didn't have the balls to tell me that I was right. I knew him better than he knew himself. I was done. I told him to talk to his daughter and handed Jakeyla the phone.

When she got off the phone, I explained to her that her dad and I were done. She looked sad but then told me of a conversation that she had overheard. She told me that her dad had picked her up and that he was on the phone with his friend. He told him that he was over to some girl's house and while she was at work, he was snooping and saw her bank statement. She had about $10,000 in the bank and he was going to be with her in order to get some of that. He said that she was buying a house and they were going to move. Wow! He was so disrespectful to be talking about his infidelities in front of our daughter. I told Jakeyla that everything will be okay. I never told him about this, but this was the straw that broke the camel's back. He was with Dawn, the one he had a child with while we were married. They got married and karma did visit the home. I am not happy about her going through what I did, but she actually thought that he would be faithful.

I had to show my daughter that this is not an acceptable relationship. I had to show her that her mother was stronger without him. The things that were displayed in the presence of my child are the things that she will learn. I had done enough by letting him come back over and over again knowing that he was poison to my life.

I wouldn't answer any of his calls to the house. He started calling the kids, family members and friends looking for me. He would leave threats too, but it was funny to me because he was so certain that I would still be waiting on him. I told him that we needed to close the chapter of this book because it was time for it to end. He thought I was playing. He was so caught up in himself that if I did ask him for something for our daughter Jakeyla, that he thought it was a plot. So, guess what? I stopped asking. He went so far as to tell people that he was doing for Jakeyla and that I was lying. I would never use my daughter to get anything from someone. But because he is such a liar and manipulator, he assumed everyone else was too. Eventually, everyone saw the things he lied about and who he truly was. I was just hurt that Jakeyla had to find out about her dad. The woman he was with was so insecure about me, but she did not have to be. I already had what she got and I was not trying to get it back. As a matter of fact, I started to write her a letter a couple of times to thank her for not giving up on her dream of having him.

The separation was extremely hard on Jakeyla and me. Jakeyla was missing her dad. But mostly she was beginning to resent him for not being there for her. I did all I could to make her happy. He would tell her that he would come get her and he wouldn't show up or bring the other child when he did come to get her. I did not have anything against the child.

Jakeyla and I grew closer. We trusted each other. My stepson, Ladarius, was an important asset to my life as he became a man. He began taking on the responsibilities of helping us. He touched my heart when he called a family meeting to tell me that I need to kick his dad to the curb. He said that I could do much better and that his dad needed to grow up. My son did whatever I needed help with in taking care of his sister. I was so proud of the man he had become. He was my son. Although the marriage wasn't a good one, I did continue to pray for my ex to be able to let us go. I wanted to be happy.

I needed to be happy. I began to enjoy myself. I gained weight, slept at nights and did not worry about what people thought anymore. At first, I was frightened when I was approached by a young man. I was feeling like I was betraying my husband although we were separated. I did give him my number and went out several times before I brought him around my daughter. I did not want her to see different people in my life. I wanted her approval of the person that I would venture with. I was enjoying myself. I was embracing the fact that I had someone that catered to me.

I did inform my ex that I was dating. He thought I was telling him a lie so he would get jealous and come back. Wait a minute! Who was asking him back? It sure wasn't me! But he thought that until his sister met the guy and went back and told him that she met my friend. He went off saying that I was disrespecting him by bringing a dude by to meet his sister. I was shocked about this response because disrespect is a word that shouldn't come out of his mouth. I quickly told him that I did not bring anyone around your sister, she came to my job and my friend was there to pick me up. I laughed at him because it was very funny. He continued trying to intervene in my dating.

The divorce was very much needed for me. Lamar really did not want to get a divorce, but it became necessary when my sister-in-law passed. He had told the woman he was living with that we were divorced. He had brought me some papers to sign but they were never filed. I am guessing he showed her those. When my name had to be on the obituary, that's when all hell broke out. His girlfriend was upset. He's been living a lie for years. Lamar texted me and said that we needed to close this chapter. I texted him back and said, "Boy don't use words that I told you years ago. It has been time for this chapter to close."

The way he came at me to get the divorce was so unexpected and pitiful. I was mad. I wasn't mad that he wanted the divorce, I was mad at how he did it. When we signed the papers, I was fine. He wanted to take me to breakfast and also wanted a hug. I wasn't mad at him, but those things were not alright with me. What were we going to talk about at breakfast? Why do you think I need a hug? I've been over this marriage.

I saw his mom and she said to me that I needed to get over her son. I looked at her and said nothing. I thought, "Lady, why do you think your son is that important in my life? He has no weight in my life." She always thought that her son was a jewel, but at this point in my life he was a pebble. I wasn't bothering him. He was bothering me. He would also show up unannounced. I called Lamar and told him what she said. I told him that I was tired of people thinking that I needed to get over you like I'm obsessed. I don't bother you. He said, "No Ma didn't…. I'm the one who needs to get over you, Jay." I said, "What!" He said, "I'm the one who needs to get over you. Jay, we were supposed to be travelling and enjoying ourselves. I wished things were different." I said, "Yeah, we could have."

He still wanted me to need him because he still needed me. I think that he thought that he wouldn't need me once he got a woman who would take care of him. He found out that he needed much more than that. I felt empowered to know that. That old saying about the grass looks greener on the other side. Well, it was green, but it wasn't the grass he was accustomed to. I could not worry about what he wanted or needed anymore, but I did need for people to stop accessing my life and giving him the power.

He got so paranoid whenever he could not see me or talk to me. He would text me in the middle of the night. The texts would say, "Jay I had a dream of you. I love you. No one will ever take your place." I used to save them to show that it was him with the obsession. But then I realized that it did not matter anymore what anyone thought. People love to keep the negativity going and if I give in to their mess the more it will persist. It was strange saying it out loud that I was divorced. I had been married for 20years. Half of my life was with the person's last name. I wasted a lot of time in something that was tearing me down slowly. It was time to let this go. It was time to move on. I had prepared for this move.

I feared a new relationship after 20 years of being married. I also knew what I didn't want. It was hard to separate other men from being like the man I was with. I would quickly stop talking to someone who showed signs of lying and cheating. I didn't want to be alone, but I did not want a messed-up relationship either. As time went by, I did date, but it was a whole lot different from back in the day. I had given half of my life to someone and did not know where to start. He made it difficult. I wasn't concerned with his happiness, but my own. I began looking for what I wanted to do with my life. I was so confused about where to start. I also wanted to make sure that it did not affect the children.

Chapter 3

Two Keys to my Heart

The keys to my heart are my daughter, Jakeyla and my stepson, James, but I call him by his middle name, Ladarius. These two have made my life worth living. They are always supportive and motivating me in whatever I decide to do. I thank God for showing me how worthy I am of these two amazing children.

I met Ladarius when he was two years old. He was a little firecracker. We hit it off when we first met. He thought I was a white woman. He told his mom that his dad was dating a white woman with green eyes. He has grown into an extraordinary young man. Although he is my stepson, I see him as my son. He treats me as a mom. When his dad and I were separated and on bad terms, he continued to live with me.

He was the Class Student Government President his last year of high school. He wanted me to attend the Awards day, but I told him that I had to work and could not get off. I wanted to surprise him. At this event. He recognized me as his mother and how he was honored to have me in his life. I was the one who was surprised. The dedication was to the three women who raised him, His mom Stephanie, his grandmother Peggy and then little old me, Jackie. His classmates and friends all knew me as his mom and said, Ms. Jackie, James really wanted you to be here, he loves you. I knew that he loved me.

James was my protector. Lamar, his dad and I were separated, and Lamar came to the house furious at me because he heard that I went out on a date. He grabbed me and Ladarius intervened and pushed Lamar back and said, "Dad, I don't want to fight you, but you are not going to put your hands on her." I was not worried about him putting his hands on me, but I was proud of my son for being a man.

Lamar was shocked. He then calms down because he realized that his son was a man and standing up for his mother. He said, Son, I am proud of you for taking up for your mother, but I will beat your bleep! Personally, I think Ladarius would have given him a good match. Meanwhile, He did not know that Jakeyla was behind him with her bat ready to swing! Did I mention that I love these kids!

Ladarius, Jakeyla and I were a family. No, we are a family. We do family meetings to inform each other of our plans, do interventions and then get advice. I remember Jakeyla telling me, dad is not going to do right. You are too good to him. They both said, we do not want you to be unhappy and you do not have to be with him because of us. I was stunned. We know about the things that you have put up with and we want you to stop putting up with this mess with him and live. I promised them that I would not allow their dad to control the situation again and I kept my promise.

I learned that no matter what you think that you are hiding from your children they see what is going on. I thought that I was making them happy. I thought that I was hiding all the pain and unhappiness. My wonderful and intelligent children were not fooled. They get it from me, their mother. They are my life, my loves and my inspiration. I always acknowledge, Stephanie, Ladarius's mother, for allowing me to be a part of his life.

On July 17, 1993, at 10:30 a.m., I gave birth to a beautiful 5lb baby girl who stole my heart. The first time I saw her I was so happy. She was my pride. Her name is

Jakeyla Sharlissa Cowlin. Her middle name came from my best friend, Melissa and Lamar's mother name, Sherry.

Jakeyla was a very smart little girl. I would not let anyone keep her that much. She stayed with my family which was my mom, grandmother or Aunt. I would call them every hour on the hour to check on her. They said I was overprotective. Maybe I was but it helped to develop a very responsible and independent woman. She was and still is my motivation. My life had so much meaning just because Jakeyla is in it. She made it easy being a mother. Everything changed in my heart and soul once Jakeyla was born. I wanted to do better and be better.

I wanted her to excel beyond all odds. Jakeyla was a very smart little girl. She was observant and inquisitive. I knew that I had to be careful of what I did in front of her. As a mother, you can still learn from your children. Jakeyla had taught me so much. She was always observant of the things that were in her surroundings. I had to be careful of what I did or showed her.

When Jakeyla was born, she was and will always be my best accomplishment. I gave birth to the most wonderful daughter a mother could have asked for. I am so proud to have given her life, instill morals and values in her, teach her what a woman does, and how to be strong and to always remember where she comes from. She taught me a BFF can be your child. Jakeyla had always been the reason I did the things I did. I went back to school to get my master's. I went back to work to provide for her. I worked three part time jobs. I made sure she did not want for anything. I was also taking care of my step niece. It was a struggle especially when my husband, and I separated. He became the father that bragged on his daughter but never participated in her accomplishments.

We bumped heads a lot. But I am the dominant one! One thing about me is that I give you credit when you deserve it. I am not going to add or take away. He would lie and make people think there was a relationship with he and Jakeyla and that I was just bitter. He had the wrong one it was your daughter honey that's bitter. I had been over it. But that was his problem. He thought that I was still taken by him and in love with him. It died years ago. I never told Jakeyla anything bad about her dad. It was all the failed promises.

When people would see me, they would inquire about my health, I would explain that I found out that I had Lupus six month after having my child. I said it so much not realizing my daughter thought that she was the reason I had

Lupus. When she told me that she was sorry, I asked for what? She said, for giving you Lupus. I said BABY, you did not give me Lupus, and I was going to have Lupus anyway. I had a doctor's appointment the next day.

Dr. Powers asked me did I have anything to live for. I sat there thinking about my daughter and said, I do, my daughter. I left his office crying and knew I had to do better. I got home and looked in the mirror and said this is not me. I do not know who she is, but she is not Jackie. That night when my daughter went to bed, I started crying. I thought that Jakeyla was sleep but she crawled over to me put my head in her little lap, kissed my head and said I hope it makes you feel better. This is something I would do to her whenever she cried or got hurt. I just cried because I got to show her strength. I wanted her to know the power of strength. I started showing that I can be strong through anything.

The Homework.

Whenever I was sick, her dad would help her with her homework. Jakeyla would come in my bedroom and ask me to check her homework after her dad had helped her. I would check it and say that it was correct. Lamar had noticed that she would ask me, and he finally asked her why she keeps asking her mom to check her homework after he already had… Jakeyla told him "Duh Daddy…because mama always calls you stupid!" He looked at me and told me that I needed to stop saying things like that to her and I told him that I didn't tell her that and that I would never do that. He told Jakeyla that he was not stupid, but she walked out of the room while saying under breath, that's not what mama tells Stephanie.

The Bat.

Jakeyla's dad bought her a bat and ball. You know the yellow bat with the white ball. She was bad about hitting people with that bat! She hit me with the bat, and I was going to whip her, but her dad stopped me. He says that little bat could not hurt you. So, I did not punish her. Later that week, I was bringing in the groceries and I saw Jakeyla walk into the bedroom and came out dragging the yellow bat. She walked into the living room where her dad was lying on the couch while talking on the phone. She swung the bat! POW! And hits her dad on the head and said I want some juicy! She dropped the bat and ran to me. Lamar came in the kitchen holding his head and said that he was going to whoop her, but I said, no you are not because that little bat could not hurt you! He got the bat and ball and threw them in the trash.

Jakeyla was still holding my leg and peeking around the corner at him.

Motherhood.

Jakeyla and I were close. Some people thought we acted like sisters. We always had each other's back. I did regret that she had to grow up helping to care of me. It was too much for a little girl. I would try to make her think that I was fine so that she would hang out with her friends. She would go but would call to check on me every hour. Eventually, she would just come home to sit with me. I have told her how sorry I was for depriving her of her childhood and then she would say, "Mama, I love you. It's my job to care for you like you care for me." I had rules in my house, and I expected them to be followed. I did not negotiate punishments. I think that rules build structure and character. My family thought that I was too strict, but I did not care. I wanted to raise a young woman that would be intelligent, independent, and respected.

I remember one time when her aunt asked if she could go to a dance, and I agreed. I told her that Jakeyla needed to be home by 11p.m. My sister said, "It's alright, she will be with me." I told her that I don't care who she is with, she needs to be home by 11p.m. I called my sister's phone at 11p.m. and she didn't answer. I called my daughter's phone and I told her to tell her aunt that she is late. Her aunt said, "It's okay, your mom knows that you are with me." I said put her on the phone. Her aunt says, "Hello." I said, "Jakeyla is late, are you bringing her home or do I need to come picks her up?" She says, "Really Jackie? She is with me." I said, "Tell Jakeyla I will call her when I get outside." And I hung up. My sister was shocked and mad.

Jakeyla had both black and white friends. The white girls would respect my rules and have her home by curfew, but the black girls would call with excuses as to why they are late. She rode to the game with some friends, and it was crowded at McDonald's so that was okay, but they called me an hour later with another excuse. I told them to come home now! Her friend comes in the house and walks in my room to explain what happened. I cut her off and told her to turn around little girl and go back out of my door and go home. She walked out with her mouth wide opened.

My daughter had started being disrespectful to her teachers because the black girls told her that she talks and acts like a white girl. That day when I had a meeting with the teacher, I was furious. I was not expecting this. I went into the classroom where the teacher began to tell me that my daughter was talking back and being disrespectful. I was in disbelief, but I was not going to jump down the teacher's throat. I could not wait to talk to Jakeyla. I was sitting there thinking that I am going to kill this little girl. Then another teacher came in and tells me of her concerns about Jakeyla. They emphasized about how she was such an intelligent little girl that they would hate to see go down a bad road. They said she has always been a very polite and obedient girl until about two weeks ago. I said her dad and I are separated, and she is close with her dad. I told them that her disrespectful ways were no excuse for her acting like this. I told them that after that day, they would NOT have this problem again, and if they did, here are my direct numbers to my line at my job, cell and house.

I walked out of that classroom ashamed and embarrassed. Jakeyla came to the car and finally her dad showed up…late. I informed him of what happened. He was shocked. I asked Jakeyla what was the problem? She told me what was said by her classmates. I rolled my eyes and said look baby girl, you do not have to be disrespectful to your elders and talk ratchet to be black. You sure as heck don't have to be stupid and dumb to be black either because you are just too smart for that. I correct you when you pronounce words incorrectly or use the incorrect noun and verb because

I want you to be educated and smart. Your true friends would want you to be the best you can be. A friend can be black, yellow, blue or orange. What you are not going to do is disrespect these teachers and not do your best. I told her that if I had to come back to that school again for that type of nonsense, then it's her and me. You are too smart to be following anyone that says you got to act a certain way to blend in. You better tell those little girls to talk to you when they get their grades up! Jakeyla's accomplishments never seemed to amaze me. She graduated from high school and college. Then she gave birth to my first grandson, who is also the love of my life. Then, she had an article in the ATL Magazine.

It goes like this:

Jakeyla, can you briefly walk us through your story – how you started and how you got to where you are today.

Graphic design has always been in my wheelhouse of talents. However, up until now, I only viewed it as a side hustle instead of a business. Since the 6th grade, my dream career has always been a psychologist. In December 2016, I received my bachelor's degree in Psychology from Auburn University (War Eagle!). Unfortunately, following graduation my mother (who has Lupus) was diagnosed with stage 4 breast cancer on January 17, 2017. I willingly paused my pursuit to go to grad school in order to focus on my mother's health (Love you, Jacks!). Thankfully, on November 30, 2018, she received the good news of being cancer free!

Through some unforeseen circumstances, I was later let go from my job. A few months down the road, I decided to make a change for the better. It took me being unemployed, depressed, lost, and newly pregnant to evaluate my course of life. Motherhood was right around the corner, so it was time to take a different approach. Although my loved ones are very supportive and never pressured me about getting a job, I desired to achieve income to support my family.

Therefore, I never planned on graphic design becoming a huge part of my life. However, Create with Key allows me to fulfill my passion for helping others apart from my original plan.

Has it been a smooth road?

My journey has not been easy. However, the circumstances I face lead me to appreciate my blessings so much more. My main two struggles have been my mother going through cancer and becoming unemployed in February 2018.

With my mother, it was as if I was watching my superhero discover her kryptonite. However, witnessing and experiencing cancer with her made me stronger. Through her, I had a front row seat to what strength looks like in human form. As a result, the experience taught me to never question my limits. Finances have been an issue as well.

Going from being able to financially support myself and my mother to not making any income was life changing. However, it humbled me and gave me the hunger to improve my situation. Sometimes, it's all about how you look at your circumstances. They can either make you or break you.

Please tell us more about your work, what you are currently focused on and most proud of.

I'm a self-taught freelance graphic designer who specializes in logos, flyers, and invitations. Although, I'm up for any challenge! My eagerness to provide each client with a satisfied product always triumphs over any obstacles I'm up against.

The amount of work and time I put into Create with Key is what makes me proudest to call it my business. I can confidently stand behind this brand because I know the countless hours, I spent building my portfolio, creating my website, studying YouTube videos, and generating a clientele. It's a huge accomplishment and a reflection of my hard work.

My customer service sets me apart from others. Helping people will always mean more to me than money, and I truly believe it shows through my customer service. I'm not satisfied until my client is 100% satisfied.

Do you have a lesson or advice you'd like to share with young women just starting out?

To young women: aligning your passions with your talents is the perfect combination that results in happiness and success! The road will get tough, but your hardships are going to be what define you. Stay resilient and know that only YOU can stop you! Make sure that you learn the lesson(s) that God intended during each season and never stop growing!

When I read this article, I was very proud of Jakeyla. She had a lot going on in her life. She did not have a good relationship with her dad, although she desperately wanted to be close with him. She was always worried about me while trying to go to college. She was a determined young woman, and I was taken by the contents in the article. She is so ambitious and always wants me to enjoy life. We have been through a lot in our lives, and I am so grateful to have Jakeyla. My marriage wasn't the best, but I would not change anything that involves Jakeyla. I genuinely believe that she is the reason for me striving to live. I never would have thought that I could love someone with all my soul. Someone that I would die for. God truly blessed me with the perfect daughter. He knew exactly what I needed in a child.

On July 9, 2018, which was my birthday, she found out that she was pregnant. I was the happiest person. I was proud to be a grandmother. After all that I had been through,

I did not think I would live to see a grandchild. So, for her to be pregnant was just another blessing that God saw that I was worthy. I was there every second. I wanted her to go through this pregnancy without any compilations or worries. I was also grateful that Kyler's father is an excellent father. He had been so incredibly supportive of Jakeyla and Kyler. Since this baby boy, Kyler Ashton McElrath has been born, my life has been so fulfilling. I find myself being full of life even on those days I am in pain or don't feel well. He comes in and gives me the biggest hugs and kisses. When he calls me Gigi, it just does something to me. Jakeyla has given me all the things I need to have to be fulfilled. I tell her often how proud I am of her and how much my life has meaning because of the love she shows me.

Ladarius and Jakeyla have been the blessings that I needed in my life. I don't know where I would be without their encouragement, support and love. I am so proud of them both. They are the reasons for me being a mother, a fighter and a survivor.

Chapter 4

Lupus: The Disease, Struggle and the Fight

In December 1993, exactly six months after I gave birth to my daughter, Jakeyla, I was diagnosed with Lupus. I was unable to take care of her properly, but I made it work. I would use all my strength to change her pamper or make a bottle. It would hurt so bad that getting up to change her, making a bottle or giving her a bath would be difficult. She was and still is my motivation to make sure she was taken care of. Being a mother made me stronger and more determined to beat this disease. I did not know much about this disease, and I did not think that it was something to worry about. I had this little girl who somehow made life seem much better and much brighter than I could ever imagine.

The kind of Lupus I have is SLE. I was not aware of this disease. I didn't think it was that serious at first. I began to let myself go.

I wasn't taking my medicines like I was supposed to, and my body would ache so bad that it hurt to cry. I would be in the bed afraid to turn because of the pain I would endure. I would just lay there trying to plan my movement. I wouldn't tell anyone because they were not familiar with the disease either therefore, they would not believe me about the things I would tell them. I would tell them of the pain in my body. My feet would swell so much that it would be unbearable to walk on them. I tried to continue working and I could not stay on the job. My feet would have this burning sensation that felt awful. I couldn't work so I tried getting help from family members who thought that I was lying or on drugs. It was even said that I just didn't want to work so I made up being in pain. Sadly, to say, my own family members told those lies. When I realized how I was lied on, I became distant. I was hurt and confused as to why I was lied on…

I tried to hide what I was going through so that I wouldn't lose my husband because I was afraid, he wouldn't understand and leave me, but I did not want him to touch me.

I kept a lot of my pain and cries to myself until one day I couldn't take it anymore. I had to call someone to take me to the Emergency Room. The ER doctor's name was Dr. Pearson. He was the one who opened the eyes of my family. He came in to talk to me and I informed him that I have Lupus and told him of the symptoms that I was having. He told my family and friends that I was a sick young lady. He goes on to tell the things that I would be going through.

I remember my grandmother saying she's been saying that, but someone told me she was on drugs. He tells her that there weren't any drugs in my system not even the drugs that I needed to be taking. She said that she promises I wouldn't be out of my medicines anymore. He gave me a shot and prescriptions. I felt better within a few days. I was glad that he told them that I was not faking an illness. I know that they didn't understand Lupus, but they should have known me better. Although he said that she would make sure I wouldn't give out anymore, I still felt like I could not trust anyone and decided to do things on my own. She did not do as much as family members thought because she barely knew if I was sick.

I lost so much weight. I could not eat anything without getting nauseous. I was at 95 pounds after giving birth… Dr. Powers saw that I wasn't following his instructions. Then, he asked me, "Do you have anything to live for young lady?" I said, "Yes sir." He said, "Well if you don't take your medicines or make your appointments, then you might live to see another Christmas." I went home thinking about what he said to me. It puzzled me. I went to the bathroom and looked in the mirror long and hard. I did not like the person that I saw. It wasn't me. I didn't know that person in the mirror. She looked like me, but the strength was gone. There was no fight in her, but there is plenty of fight in me. I had to change the path that I was on. It was taking me to a bad place.

I decided that day that I was going to do to do something different. I began eating, taking my medication and I made my appointments. I did have a few flare ups because of the stress of trying to keep it together. I was trying hard to get over obstacles. Lupus had me asking God why me? What have I done to deserve this kind of disease? It took a lot for my eyes to open to know the answers. God was testing my faith, my strength and my belief in him. Somewhere in the past. I gave up on God before Lupus. I guess when my friend was killed. I could not understand why a good person had to die…Especially to be killed. I always heard older people say that God never puts more on you than you can bare. God, am I that strong? Do you see me carrying all these problems, taking care of all these people, handling the marriage, the diseases and life?

I actually thought that Lupus was the end of my life. Consequently, it was the beginning of my life, once I began to understand it. Lupus was part of my life and I had to learn to adjust to the flare ups and know the symptoms. I started researching the disease. I wanted to control the disease. I had to convince my family that I could handle lupus. I knew that they only wanted to protect me.

I went into the hospital when Hurricane Katrina hit in Louisiana in 2008. The doctors thought that I was having a stroke because of the weakness in my left side, but it turned out that I had an infection in my spine. I stayed in the hospital for over a month. I could not walk. I had to learn how to walk again. It was a difficult time. I was in so much pain that I would be on a morphine pump the duration of my hospital stay. After I was released, my rheumatologist wanted to start a treatment called Apheresis to help me with my Lupus. Apheresis is a medical term in which the blood of a person is passed through an apparatus that separates out the constituents and returns the remainder to the circulation.

I took three of these treatments, but on the third one I never knew why I was being saved or knew that I was being saved. I just knew that it wasn't my time. I had near death experiences that allowed me to be a witness to the death of my friends. I would be the one who would identify their killers.

God saved me from two murders, two illnesses and one marriage. **His will for me to live was stronger than his destination for me to die.** I did not think that I was praiseworthy. As I lay in the hospital to take a treatment that I had taken a few times before, I began to feel my airways closing. I tell the nurse who is administering my treatment of my airways feeling like it was closing. She pushes the call button. I quickly call my aunt who would normally be home. She did not answer. I was panicking. I knew everyone else was at work. I called Kiki, my best friend's daughter. She answered and I tell her to call everyone to let them know what happened. Yeah, I know…Where was the husband? Well, he was with the other woman and no it was not discussed with the family.

A bunch of nurses rushed in and started taking out tubes. One of the tubes was in my neck and the nurse forgot to clamp it off and blood was everywhere. I heard a code blue, and I woke up in CCU (Critical Care Unit). While I was out, a vision came to me and said that it was not my time, and that God has a plan for me. I had to go back to do what he has for me. I asked what is it that I need to do. She said you will know it when he shows you. I woke up with body aches everywhere. My back was bruised. I was taken downstairs for some tests, and it was cold, and it took a long time. When I returned upstairs, my doctor was in the hallway, and he was asking questions about why my nurse wasn't escorting me to these tests. He started cursing her out.

I didn't know how long I was in CCU, but all my family and friends were there. When I saw my sister, Inger, I started crying and I asked her if I was dying? She told me no and I asked if she was sure because Popeye (my other sister) doesn't get off work for anything and they just laughed. Apparently, I had a reaction to the treatment and could not receive the treatment anymore. I laid there thinking about what happened in the dream. Does God have a plan for me, and if he does what is it? I was anxiously waiting on the message from him.

My nurse saw that I was awake and told me that I had an important phone call. There wasn't a phone in the room, so I had to be moved to the desk to take the call. I answered and it was my husband. I hadn't talked to this man in two or three weeks. He had lied to the nurse saying that he was in the army overseas when he got the call. I was furious! I was so angry that my blood pressure was high.

When I was finally put into a room, I sat there and did a lot of thinking. I realized that people that I thought would be supportive by calling or showing up, didn't. I was so hurt and promised myself that I wasn't going to allow it to bother me. I became stronger after this episode. I could not believe that the people who I thought the most of was not there. I had this dream while I was out of it, this person was telling me that it was not my time, and that God has a plan for me and that I am not done here. It seemed so real. I could not stop thinking of those words… "God has a plan for you." What plans? He isn't through with me?

I had a follow up with my doctor and this lady came and sat by me and said, "You know you have a gift, and you should use it. You know things about people, but you don't say anything. What God is showing you are the ones who you need to help and who you need to be careful with. Trust yourself." I just smiled and nodded. I didn't know her. Was this real? She knew things that I had not spoken to anyone.

While I was in the hospital, a family member came to visit. They said that the reason I was in this situation was because I don't go to church. I was like, Wow! Really? I could not believe the words that came out of their mouth! I began asking that person if the Deacons who are in church every Sunday that leave to go to the bootleggers have more faith than me. I said you mean to tell me that the ones in church every Sunday that speak to you in church but turn their heads in the street has more faith than me? I asked them if they were saying that God favors them because they come to church every Sunday…Well, let me tell you this, (I said) …I have more faith than anyone because of what I've been through because you see He brought me through it. I don't have to be in church every Sunday to be grateful or to give God praise in front of others in order for God to know that I believe in Him or have faith in Him. I would have thought that you of all people would come here to encourage and inspire me, instead of discouraging me.

The family member did not say a word but left the room. I called my mom to tell her about the conversation just so she would be prepared. I realized that God dictates our lives through the things that He allows us to go through. The test is for you to pass so that you can get to what He has for you. ***Never let anyone think that because you do not attend***

church every Sunday, that your praise, and faith is not strong or worthy. I used to be ashamed to go to church if I hadn't been in a while; But I know that I give God all of me. I don't have to prove to anyone the level of my faith or my relationship with God! I thought that I wasn't worshiping Him because I was not doing the things that the others were doing in church. I could not follow the members because my worship is my own individual kind. Sometimes the words of a song just hit me with spirit, and I shed tears. I know that the spirit doesn't have to hit you just in church because if you are filled with the Holy Ghost, it can be anywhere. How can a person say something like this just because they don't go to church?

I started keeping to myself. I was reluctant in telling anyone if I was sick. I didn't want to bother them. I didn't want pity. I would deal with the pain alone. It was hard, but I managed. I was told about how people were talking about me, and those same people would be the ones that I would help. I did not tell them of what I was told, and I did not treat them any different either. I thought family was supposed to be for you and not jealous or envious of you. I learned that blood does not necessary means closeness or loyalty. Some family can be just as devious as snakes.

I had to realize that I needed to take care of me. I knew that I needed to get rest, but it seemed to be impossible. I was always focusing on others and depriving myself of the things that I needed to do. I would always want to be that person who everyone needed. I also wanted someone that I could lean on as well. I became so caught up in trying to please others that I forgot about the one that really needed help, me.

Although Lupus was tough to deal with, it taught me a lot. I learned to be patient, to be strong and to be encouraged. I had to take care of me because no one else was going to do it and I had to be aware of what was going on. I began to be overwhelmed with guilt that I was putting it on the people that I love. I knew no one would understand what I was going through and did not let them know unless it became so unbearable that I could not handle it. I was afraid to lose my husband even though he wasn't good for me. He was toxic. I was in love with him no matter what he had done or was doing. I finally realized that I was in love by myself. I was married but alone. I thought daily about how I would leave him. When I started thinking of ways to hurt him physically, I knew that I needed to get out of the relationship. I was tired of the mental abuse. I was tired of him feeling pity for me. I did not need that. I needed for him to respect me or at least love me enough to want to not hurt me or cause any pain to the woman who was always there for him.

I was always stressing over what everyone thought or how people would perceive me as being helpless. That's why nobody ever seen me hurting but smiling. They never knew that I was struggling but surviving. They never knew that I knew they talked about me, and they thought we were still cool. I could not be broken anymore. I had become too strong to let my heart, soul and faith be broken. God had shown me that I was one of His warriors.

Chapter 5

Cancer: The Treatments, The Depression and the Survival

Facebook Post: 1/24/18

I am one of those people who must do better with patience. When I started Chemo, I was in a hurry to get Chemo done. But my daughter, Jakeyla Cowlin had to remind me that I had to be patient. My hair started falling out then I wanted to get it cut. I wanted it to grow back. Now that it's growing back, I'm getting impatient because it's not growing back like I want. I kept getting this bill about my account and I'm knowing it was paid but I kept calling, but calls weren't returned. I get an email saying that it has been taken cared of except a small amount. But today, I realized that when you pray for things, they come as God has planned. I must be patient and be still.

I was feeling myself becoming depressed. I felt like I wasn't going to make it. I tried extremely hard not to let my family see this scary part of my struggle. It wasn't that I was giving up, it was because of the things that Cancer was taking me through. My cousin, Arianna was diagnosed with stage 4 stomach cancer. She was diagnosed before I was. I would call to keep check on her and she would check on me too. Whenever she called me, we would talk about how people don't understand about the eating habits or the things we were experiencing. The hurtful part is that she was in Stage 4 and there wasn't anything they could do but make her comfortable. She was strong throughout it all. When she passed on August 2, 2017, I was so hurt for her daughter and her sisters.

I prayed for my family to have strength to help them to accept whatever God has planned for me. Cancer was more intense and threatening. I don't know exactly when I noticed the lump in my breast, but it was after I got over the shingles by the way is very painful. I had just got over the shingles and started having pain in my breast. It was hard and sore to touch. I felt like I was being torched whenever I wore a bra. I mentioned it to my daughter, and she told me that I needed to make an appointment to get a mammogram. I couldn't remember the last time that I had seen an

OB/GYN. I tried to contact my doctor, but she no longer took my insurance. I googled OB/GYN doctors that took my insurance at Brookwood hospital so that all my doctors could be in the same place. I managed to get in touch with one and I was incredibly pleased with my choice. Before she examined me, she had her nurse to seat me in her office. She came into the office, and we discussed what was going on with me. She told me that she was going to run tests to see what could be going on. I had other concerns but the lump in my breast was priority. As she was examining me, she explained the different scenarios of what could be going on, but she didn't confirm any of them until she ran the tests.

After examination, she sent me to get a mammogram immediately. Before I left, Dr. Taylor wanted to say a prayer with me, and I felt safe to accept her prayer. I went to do my mammogram. This was the most painful mammogram I've ever had in my life. She kept squeezing my breast. I had tears in my eyes. The technician kept apologizing for hurting me, but I told her that I was okay. I told her to just continue doing her job so that the tests would be accurate. When we were done testing, she told me to go sit in the waiting area while she called the doctor. I had this feeling that something was wrong. I had an unnerving feeling. I sat there like she asked but I was in a lot of pain.

As I was sitting there, so many things were going through my head, and I was preparing myself for whatever it was. The technician came back and said that the doctor had gone into surgery so they would call me. I said ok and left still with a million things going through my mind. I began to get myself together for whatever fight that I was about to go through. I did not know exactly but I felt like it was going to be some type of battle.

When I realized that I might be in a situation where Jakeyla could possibly have only one parent, I called Lamar to talk to him about trying to rekindle and build a relationship with her. But the conversation ended with me telling him to not call me for anything and we were completely done. He did not want this to happen. He even said I was wrong, but I felt the same about him. I wanted him to do this before he found out that something was happening to me. So, I blocked his phone calls.

The relationship with him and Jakeyla was dead. He wasn't realizing that he has hurt her in so many ways with disappointments. I had been trying for a while to get them into a relationship but one (Jakeyla) wasn't hearing it and the other one (Lamar) was living in a fantasy thinking that they were good. He would call her to ask to ask if they could spend the day together but would invite his outside child along with them. Jakeyla felt like he was depriving her of time with her dad and he could not see this. No matter how hard that I tried to tell him the more we argued. I got tired and I let it go. I was finished and so was Jakeyla. He needed me, but everyone thought that I needed him.

When I got home, I called my family and told them that I was waiting for the results. My family was more concerned with the results than I was. I get a call the very next day to meet with the surgeon to see about getting a biopsy. He scheduled me the next day, so I asked my friend, Stephanie, to ride with me. She said yes without hesitation. I called to inform my family about my appointment, and they told me to let them know what the doctor said.

We arrived at the surgeon's office, and they called me back. He came in to talk to me and told me that he wanted to examine me. I asked Stephanie if she wanted to stay while they examine me, and she said sure. While he was examining me, I was making sounds to indicate that it hurts, and he was apologizing. He told me that he wanted to do a biopsy and I said okay. He then told me that he would have to do it today right here in this office. I looked at Stephanie. I was surprised, but I said okay. They prepared me for the biopsy.

Stephanie stayed during the whole process. I was so glad for her to be there because it was unexpected. He explained that I would be sore and that the area where he took the specimen from would be black and blue. It happened just as he described. I called my mother to tell her that the doctor was doing the biopsy. She thought that I knew about the biopsy, but I didn't know that he was going to the biopsy in his office. Dr. Littleton told me that he would contact me once the results are back, and I said okay. Stephanie told me in the car that we are going to pray about this. I said okay but I still had this uneasiness about everything. She kept telling me that "We" got this. I liked that statement because all my closest friends said that exact word, "We".

On January 17, 2017, around 4:30 pm, my daughter called me to see if I had gotten my results. I tell her no, but I will call you as soon as I find out. Later that night, I got a call from my daughter, Jakeyla, asking me if they had called me about the results. Then she says some words that tore my heart to pieces not for me but for her. She said they called me with your results. Apparently, they thought I was you. I said what was it? She starts crying and I knew. They said that you are positive for breast cancer. She cried even harder. I said to her, “Baby, I will be okay.” I know you are hurting but I need for you to calm down and tell me exactly what they said so I can know what I have to do. She told me that I had come call his office to schedule an appointment the next day. I say okay. I talked to her until she was calm. I wanted to take that pain from my baby. This was not the way she should have found out. I told her to get herself together and that I would call her back. She said, “Okay". I said, "I love you!" She tells me that she loves me too. I turned the car around to go back to my mother's house to tell them. My baby sister, Shaquanda, was leaving so I told her that I got my results back. She said, "What is it?" I said, “I'm positive for Breast Cancer." with a smile on my face. She said sadly, "Oh!" and got in her car.

I went in the house to tell my parents. I told my mother, but my stepdad wasn't there. The look in her eyes told me that she had already given up on me. She thought of Cancer as a death sentence. I told her that I am going to be okay. I don't think she believed me. I got in the car to call my sister, Inger, who was at a basketball game. I kept calling her, she finally picked up. I told her of my results. She said, "I'm leaving the game now. I'll call you back!" I was worried that she was crying, and people would notice her because we are light complexion, and our face turns red when we cry. Next, was my brother, Robert. I called him and he was so quiet. I said "Hey!” He said very softly, "I'm here." I tell him that he can call me back whenever he wanted to talk. He said, “Okay". I called my stepson, Ladarius, but he did not answer so I texted him to call me. The last call was to my aunt Lessie. When I told her, she didn't hold back her tears like everyone else. She started crying. I told each of them not to be worried. I asked my family not to tell anyone about me having Cancer. I did not want anyone outside my family to know. I felt like they would think of me as poor Jackie, she already has Lupus and now Cancer. I finally called my friend Stephanie to tell her. She said not to worry because we are going to beat this thing my friend. I talked to her for hours which weren’t unusual for us. I got off the phone and called my daughter back to check on her. She was not feeling well but thank God for her line sisters of Delta Sigma Theta because they were right there for her. The next day, I called Dr. Littleton's office and he scheduled me an appointment for the day after.

All of my family came to support me except my mom because she had to have surgery, but my aunt went in her place. I went to the appointment with my family which was the entire waiting room. They called me back but only two could come to the back with me, so my sisters came. My doctor came in and said that I had other family members out there that wanted to come in and if it was okay for them to come back…I said, "Yes sir." The remainder of my family and friends came in to listen to what Dr. Littleton was going to say about the plan. They all came in to hear the results. He told me that I had Stage 3A Breast Cancer. I took a deep breath and heard sniffling amongst my sisters and aunt. I looked at them with positivity and strength. My brother looked sad. I've never seen him this way. Dr. Littleton tells me of the appointment he has scheduled for me with an Oncologist, Dr. Ashraft.

Dr. Littleton would put in my port. The port will be used to give me my chemo treatments. Dr. Ashraft would take care of the treatments. I saw Dr. Ashraft, and he told me of how many treatments I would take and the possibility of radiation. My family was very hurt. They tried not to let me see them cry, but I was okay with it. He showed us the size of the Cancer. Shaquanda, my baby sister, was in complete tears by now. My sister, Inger, and Aunt Lessie was also shedding tears.

My brother was calm but had a look of worry. I asked a couple of questions and Stephanie asked questions too. When we left the office, I started conversations to get their minds off what had happened. My aunt wanted me to live with her during my treatments. Everyone agreed. While they were laughing and talking about my brother's driving, I was texting my other brother, Raman, on my dad's side. I told him about the diagnosis. He responded with Dam! Dam! I was trying to text him back, but he was calling so I answered. He said, "I said, Man she has Lupus too! Why her!" I told him that I'm going to be okay. He tells me to keep him posted and I told him that I would. We said that we loved one another and hung up. I was overjoyed with his response and call. I wanted a relationship with him.

We lost our dad two years prior to me getting my diagnosis. When we got home, we had to tell my mother of what the doctor discussed with us. My mom was a mess. She was upset. To her, I was her baby although I was the oldest. I felt her pain and tried to reassure her that I was going to be okay. She didn't believe me. I can tell by the look in her eyes. My family is close knit, and we all talk every day sometimes three to four times a day. My mom, aunt, daughter, brother and sisters called me every day. That part didn't just start when they found out about me having Cancer. I love that about my family. I was scheduled to have my port in on January 26, 2017.

My son finally called back a week later and he was crying and upset. Later that day my ex-husband called. He never said he knew but I knew he knew. I knew my son had told him. I was upset with Lamar, but I answered his questions dryly. Eventually, I told him that I had to go. My cousin, Tabitha called and wanted us to pray together and fast together.

On January 21, 2017, I decided to go to church to surprise my mother. I called my sister Inger and told her to pick me up, but not to tell mama that I was coming to their church. It was crowded when we arrived, so we had to sit up front in the corner. I was okay with sitting up front. When church began, a member leaned over and said, "Jackie, you are going to be okay." I was confused as to why he said that. I think the Prophetess was preaching that day. Another member was doing the introduction and she was saying some inspirational words and looking my way. I was thinking that I'm just paranoid about thinking that someone has told them something. I said to myself, "Naw." As the service went on, I was in the spirit and clapping.

My mom came inside to usher and saw us. She had a smile on her face, and I smiled back at her. Prophetess was doing her sermon and a few times she looked my way, but I didn't find it strange. Inger bumped me and I turned to look at her. She was pointing and I couldn't see where she was pointing so I said, "What?" She said, “No, wants you." (We called our stepdad No, short for Nolan). By now, I am sure that the church knows so I am terribly upset. He motions for me to go to the altar and now I’m furious. I had asked everyone not to tell anyone. I stood there for a moment. I started to walk out but I went to the altar. Prophetess is saying something, but I wasn’t listening. I was angry but focusing on my mother who was standing at the doorway. She was crying. She walks over to me, and I hugged her tightly and whispered to her that everything will be alright, and I love you. She hugged me tightly. At that moment nothing in that church mattered except my mom.

Afterwards, I got back where Inger was sitting. I asked her who told the church. She quickly responded that it was not her. We later deduce that it was my stepdad because Inger or my mom had not been to church since I told them that I had Breast Cancer. That was three weeks prior. Inger knew I was mad. Two days later at my parents, my stepdad tells me that Prophetess said to tell you to stop running. I didn't say a word, but I was sitting there thinking, "Running? What?" I shook my head. Therefore, I did not want anyone to know about the Cancer because of all kinds of the suggestions that will be offered. I was different in a lot of cases, but similar. The results are different for me. Did she think that I was running from God or Cancer? The message was so vague. But I did not shy away from the idea. I kept having dreams of different people, but the same thing was said in the dream. It was three dreams with three people who all were deceased. They kept telling me that God wants me to tell my story. He needed for me to give my testimony.

The fight began with Cancer when I started my first Chemo on February 6, 2017. My sisters took me to my appointment. They stayed during the entire treatment. I was in a private room. It had a television, snacks and drinks for patients. It was kind of scary because I didn't know what to expect. I got through the treatment fine. I had my sisters to drop me off to meet my friend, Donna to get my hair cut low we also we hung out for a little while. Dr. Ashraft's nurses kept calling to check on me. I told them that I'm doing fine. This went on for about three days.

On the fourth day, I could not get out of the bed. I felt like my body was glued to the bed. I felt weak, and nauseous. I just had enough strength to call Dr. Ashraft's office. I told them that I was feeling awful. They told me to come to the office as soon as possible. I said that I would. I called Inger to tell her that I felt bad and must go to the doctor office. She said she would be over. I got up to get ready, but it was very hard. My Aunt had to come in to help me. Then my mother arrived to help and by that time, Inger finally arrived. They helped me in the car and my mom and aunt were crying when as we left. We met Shaquanda at her apartment. She picked up Donna and drove us to the hospital. We got there and I was so weak that I could barely walk. I gave blood and went back to the room to see the doctor.

Dr. Ashraft told me that he was going to be honest with me. He goes on to say that the insurance company would not approve the Neulasta that I needed until I got sick. They got me a wheelchair. As I sat there, they told me that I need fluids because my white blood cell count is low, and they are going to admit me to the hospital. My sisters got on their cell to call everybody. I was taken care of in the Cancer Center by Dr. Ashraft's office. They gave me fluids until the paperwork was finished.

A staff member named Kristy came in to tell me that my insurance would not approve me to be admitted into the hospital where my doctor has access. I had to go to another hospital across town. Kristy called the other hospital, but they informed her that my doctor has no authorization at their hospital to have someone admitted and that I would have to go to the Emergency Room. My sisters took me to

St. Vincent hospital, and it was crowded. It took seven hours before I was called back. I remained calm but my family was getting impatient. After waiting for hours, I was sent home feeling worse than I was before. I called Dr. Ashraft's office to tell him that I wasn't admitted into the hospital and that they sent me home. He asked if I could come to his office to get fluids. I told him that I would be there. When we arrived, I was told that I had to be given fluids in the office until the insurance approved the shot that I needed. The nurse was making arrangements. When we called to tell my mom and aunt, they were crying because they were confused with Home Health and Hospice.

I knew that they would confuse the two because they were so emotional at this point. We had to stress that they are not the same. I got the call from Home Health to arrange for services. They explained what they do and what is expected. Next, she tells me the fee is $350 to which I don't have, and I had to tell her that I would have to call her back. My sister asked what the fee was. I told her that I don't have $350. Inger says, “Here! Give them my card number.” I said to her that you just got laid off. She told me not to worry about that. I called and paid it.

They came out the next day and I got my fluids. I started to feel better. This really touched my heart that my sister would do that for me without hesitation. I went back to see Dr. Ashraft because he wanted to see me. I signed in and then got called back up for copay. I said, "I have to pay copay even if he called me in?" She said, “Yes ma’am you pay a copay every time you see the doctor." I said, "Well can I see the nurse?" She said it will still be a copay. Wow! $45 a visit to each specialist added up to $135 - $180 per week. It was such a headache. I swapped insurance which made my deductibles start over. The appointments were getting to be every week and I had to make them. Humana finally approved of me getting the Neulasta. It was a rough moment, but God arranged for all my family to be available. My daughter had just finished at Auburn University; She had a mix up with her classes which put her graduation back to December.

My sister, Inger, got laid off and my sister Shaquanda was off for a while for her surgery and mom had surgery too. It was all God's plan. It was harder on my mother than any of them, because she could not make my appointments. I called Dr. Littleton's office the next day. He scheduled me an appointment the very next day. Everyone came with me except my mom because she had surgery. My mom would apologize for not being able to come. I would tell her that it is okay because she would have to care for herself. She would always be in tears when we left for the doctor, feeling helpless. This would sadden me, but I could not be weak, I had to be strong. I had to let her know that she raised a fighter. I wanted this part of my life to be over. Instead, I had to wait patiently. After the first treatment, I was in the hospital almost after every treatment.

My white blood cell counts were low. I would have to get about three blood transfusions which I hated, but it helped. The treatments had gotten where I was vomiting and had diarrhea consistently. I was miserable because I could not eat anything. I could not sleep either because I was in so much pain along with the vomiting and diarrhea. Most of the day and nights I spent on the toilet with a trash can in front of me. I did not want to leave the house at this point because my hair was falling out. My body looked like a skeleton. I was ashamed of my body. I was ashamed of me. I did not like what I was becoming. I would look at the mirror and feel so much anger because I could have done better for myself. I was in a world that nobody knew or understood although they tried.

People would tell my family what they did or what would do but I was different, and I am different. I had to repeat that I was different, I have Lupus too. My body is different. Some of the things did help like the popsicles. I could eat those. It was hard to keep a box around. Everything else tasted awful and had me gagging. I couldn't eat food with spices, seasoning and sauces. My foods would have a bad taste and had to be cooked plain, this was the only way I could eat but not much. I could barely eat a happy meal. One bite and three fries would fill me up. That was enough. I could eat fruits better. I started eating those frequently. I had people to bring me all kinds of food that I wanted to eat. I was getting Ensure and Boost Milk, but I could not hold that down either. I was so overwhelmed with what I needed to do.

I would almost fallout with my family because they would fuss about some of the things that I could not help. Cancer makes you feel like you don't have a way out. Some days that's how Cancer had me feeling. I already was feeling helpless because my family had to help me with things that I should have been able to do myself but couldn't. They had no idea of how bad I felt about that. One time I could not make it to the bathroom, and I vomited all over the floor. My cousin Shelia came to help me clean it up without hesitation.

I felt ashamed. I kept thanking her. She told me that it was okay. But to me it was not okay. The treatments seemed to get harder and harder, but my support system got stronger and stronger. After each Chemo treatment I was admitted into the hospital because of my white blood cell count being low. It was so lonely at times.

My daughter would call constantly. She wanted to be there, but she had just got a promotion and couldn't take off. She would FaceTime to see me or to hear what the doctors were doing. Just seeing or hearing her voice would get me through the day, hour, minute or second. I would be in the hospital from three to six days, and it would be so depressing because I was limited. I couldn't go to the bathroom by myself because I was at risk of falling. There were times that the nurses would be so slow about coming so I would go to the bathroom on my own. I was so afraid, but I was not going to give up on my life. I would even be scared to sleep, so I would stay up when I was at home but tried to sleep when I was in the hospital. I couldn't get any sleep in the hospital. I would feel helpless.

The diarrhea was so horrible that I would be scared that I would mess on myself if I went to sleep. I was a mess. The nights were long. My daughter, mom, sisters, brother, friend and Aunt would call every day. Some days I did not want to talk to people. I refrained from crying, but I had thoughts about where this is going like, “Am I going to be okay?” The pain, unable to sleep, vomiting and diarrhea were all so intense. I know I am strong, but my weakness was thinking about my daughter...Will she be okay? I wanted to leave her with something to be proud of, so I began writing my testimony. I would be on Facebook and write my thoughts or things I was going through and BAM! I would get an inbox from people who are touched by something I said. Then I asked God, “Is this what I’m here for?”

I could not get my treatment and I was very upset. I also had an appointment to get a wig at the American Cancer Society. My hair had fallen out and it looked bad. It was in patches. Every time I look at my head, I got depressed. My sister took me by the American Society for my appointment. I tried on wigs and I was not happy. I felt like this is not me. I don’t look right. I took one of the wigs and some of the caps they had. I told my sister to take me to the barbershop. I decided that I would go ahead and get it all cut off. I sat in the chair, took off my scarf, and told the barber, who was a woman, I want to cut it all off. As I sat there thinking about what’s about to happen, I heard my sister sniffling. I said, “Oh my, do I look bad?” I hear the clippers buzzing and I see the fuzz falling. The buzzing stops and she wings me around to look in the mirror. I looked in the mirror and say, "Wow! I don't look bad. I am actually cute." I looked over at my sister and I see her eyes are red. I tell her that I feel better. I never wore that wig that I got from the American Cancer Society. I began to embrace my bald head. I got a lot of compliments and encouragement.

One day I was leaving a treatment and my sister stopped by Publix, normally she stays behind me but this day, she was in front of me. I was checking out and I swiped my card. I saw the cashier looking and I said, "Dang! I don't know why Shaquanda left me." I thought my card had declined. I asked the cashier, "Did my card decline?" She said, "No." The cashier started crying and said, "You are so beautiful, and I just wanted to tell you to be strong. Can I give you a hug?" I am standing there saying to myself, "Lady I thought my card was declined and you over here crying." I said yes and she called her manager to look at me. At first, I didn't know how to take it but then I realized she was just being concerned. I left and my sister asked me what happened. I tell her and she started to cry…Lord!

That day my test of faith was put to the test...I got to my appointment and the balance was behind, but I didn't worry because I know payments had been made faithfully. My blood pressure was 167/102. I didn't worry because I knew worrying would increase it…I already knew pain was the cause. When they removed my access to my port for me to leave, two things happened…Blood was shooting out and I was asked if I was on blood thinners (I answered calmly with "no") and a phone call came in the Cancer center and I overheard the nurse say they are flushing her now. There was a long pause. She got off the phone and I asked if that call was about me. She said it was and that they need to recheck my blood pressure. I said OK while still remaining calm. I texted my daughter and my sisters about what was happening. She placed the cuff on my arm. I felt it getting tighter and tighter. When it beeped, I asked if it was high. She told me yes, 176/109. I said, "oh."

By then my undershirt was covered in blood. I removed it while they tried to clean it with peroxide (a good tip) and the other nurse informed the doctor that it was high. He said keep her while we get her some medicine. So, this text comes in from none other than my baby sister, Shaquanda Coleman: OMG! You need to sit down and get some rest! I giggled… Because I knew it. Then my baby girl Jakeyla Cowlin texts coming in multiples…I had several messages when I got to my phone! Texts like, "Why is it high?" and "What's the deadline on the bill?" … I smiled. Meanwhile I'm texting my nephew, Jay Vincent, to inform him that we got to stay a little while longer. He said, "Okay Jack Jack!" I smiled. The nurse wrote my blood pressure down for me, told me to monitor my blood pressure and to get some rest.

I had neglected getting my annual mammogram because "I was too busy". I am one of the lucky…no…. blessed ones that got Cancer in order to beat it. Although I had been dealing with Lupus for 25 years, I thought that I could handle Cancer, but that battle was different. Cancer changed my body. I lost my hair, weight, and breasts. Everything I had valued in being a woman. I didn't feel like a woman at first. I was scared that I wouldn't find a companion to share my life with after losing these things. It took me a while to realize that I am still a beautiful woman and that a true man will know that by my character.

When I came home to regroup from being at the hospital with my sister, my doctor called me. I had it on Bluetooth, so it was answered through the radio. He said, "Mrs. Cowlin, your x-ray shows something in the left side where you are having pain and I know this is the area where you had Cancer." I hear my mom sniffling. I said,

"Okay." He then said, "I'm sending you to do a CT Scan." I said, "Okay." I got off the phone and turned to my mom and said, "Mama don't you get scared or think it's Cancer…It could be inflammation. Don't cry." I thought to myself, "Damn!". I didn't tell anyone yet because I didn't want anyone to worry. My family already had a lot on their plates. I got the CT scan and it confirmed that it was something there. They called and scheduled me for a PET scan. I didn't know what was going on, but my faith and loyalty was in God. I knew that he always had me and that I got this testimony to finish. God has been telling me something and I know now that I have got to get up on this platform to speak about His grace.

Chapter 6

Walk in My Shoes

Someone will always have a situation that they are given to experience. And it seems like some people who are not in that particular situation will have their own opinions and advice about your situation. I never understood why some people are always judging and soliciting their point of views without considering what if the shoe was on the other foot. In some situations, helping someone can cause people to bite the hands that fed them.

Daddy Lesson

I have always been the person who tries to keep the family active. My dad was the first man to break my heart. He got married and then he basically forgot about us, unless something happens, then he shows up. At one point I was trying extremely hard to get him to be a part of our lives. As I got older, I had resentment because of his lack in parenthood. I get that he was young when I was born and if he felt that he could not be a father, then he should not have brought three children into this world. Some of his family looked up to him and thought that he was the best dad in the world. He would come home and pass through my city and I wouldn't know it until someone asked me how long your dad has been here. I would tell them I don't know because I didn't know he was home. It was embarrassing and it hurt. I still love my dad despite the neglect. I wanted his approval.

Dad would brag about my little brother that he had with my stepmother. I did not hold that against my brother because he and I were good. I was hospitalized and he came home and visited me all of about 30 minutes. I got mad at my mom for telling my aunt to tell him that I was sick. I felt like it was a show, and that he didn't care about us. We often bumped heads because I was not impressed by him. I wanted that life with both parents, and I later realized that my stepfather stepped into our lives being that dad. He would make sure we were okay and then he adopted the three of us. My dad did not put up a fight to have us as his kids. He was more worried about the allotment that was being taken out of his check. My brother was very salty about this situation. He thought that our stepmother didn't like us. Later, I thought the same thing.

Dad did not take up for us whenever there was a situation with our stepmom. He had a heart attack, and she did not notify us until three days of him being in the hospital. We did not owe him to be by his side, but we tried to make sure he was taken care of. I was very upset that we were not told until three days later. As my sister, Inger and I are driving to check on him, she then tells me that he had been in the hospital, I decided to google the directions to the hospital to go there instead of meeting her, my husband said, so you are just going to leave her hanging, I said, yes just like she left us hanging, I called the hospital and got all the information to go see dad. She finally arrived. While we are sitting there, she tells me that she told my dad that if he was in bad shape, she would take him to the nursing home near us for us to see him. I turned liked the exorcist to look at her and said, he does not have to go into a nursing home, I'll come and get him. I did not find this funny especially when you did not tell us about our dad.

When I went back to see our dad, he told us that he drove himself to the hospital while having chest pains. I told him that he needs to add one of us to his call list so if anything happens, we will know. He added me, but she didn't know until he had another stroke. He came home for a funeral and then another family member passed. Dad was home for his brother-in-law and nephew's funeral, but the day before the funeral he had a stroke. My aunt called us to be there for him. We drove four hours to be there for him. My stepmom came the next day. I drove every day to be by his side until they took him to Georgia, I told him that I would come over to help take care of him.

I did go over to help take care of him. It was a mess. Dad got depressed because the people he was coming home to see was not checking on him for three months. He said that his sister hasn't called him since he had the stroke. I told him this is when you find out who is on your side. He said he started to jump down the flight of stairs to end his life. I told him what if it didn't end his life and he ended up in more pain. I will never let the absence of a person make me think about ways to end my life. I've had a bad marriage, trifling friend and family that would be jealous, talk about me and tell lies but I have never let them get in my head and make me think of harming myself. On the other hand, I have thought about harming them but then I realized that it's not worth it.

My dad started to cry and apologized about how he treated us. He said that he never would have thought that I would be the one to take care of him. I told him I didn't either. I was thinking that God made me a better person because I use to be bitter against my dad. I have learned throughout life that I must be a blessing to people that taught me a lesson about what was wrong in my life. He loved his sister. She was the one he would come home to visit. Dad realized that the people he was giving his time to didn't have time for him, but his kids would always be right there whenever he was down…Although he didn't have time for his kids.

Dad was not looking like himself. He needed a haircut and a shave. So, I told him that I would take him to his barber, and he was excited. My stepmom was cutting his hair with scissors. Dad's hair was too short for scissors. We went to his barber and the guy asked Dad, who was this beautiful young lady? He told him that I am his daughter. The barber asked him how many children he had, and my dad said four. The barber said that he thought he just had the one son that was in the military. Then, something hit me, and I was hurt all over again. I came here to help you and you didn't acknowledge me? I am your first born. I am the oldest and you forgot to mention me or my siblings. I started to leave him there and go back home. On the way to his house, it was quiet. I didn't know what to say to him. All I knew is that I was hurt. I don't think he knew I was hurting. I continued to stay, but it became uncomfortable.

Dad wasn't feeling well so I took him to the doctor. My stepmother was upset that I took him without letting her know. I couldn't believe her...She didn't tell me...She told dad. He got sick again and I was getting ready to take him back to the ER. He told me that Mary, my stepmom, was upset when I took him the last time. I asked him what's her number at work. He did not know it...I googled it and got her line. I told her who I was and told her that dad wasn't feeling well and that he said she was upset that I didn't call her. She asked me how I got her number and I was livid. I told her google. She told me that she would make him an appointment the next morning and I said okay. I was too mad. I knew dad wasn't going if she wasn't. I could not sleep for being mad. The thing that she should have asked was if there was anything wrong.

After this incident everything was awkward. She did make dad an appointment. We went to the appointment, but the doctor did not acknowledge her because dad told him that she stopped his blood thinners. The doctor was furious because dad needed to take them for the rest of his life. So, at the appointment, I was playing casino on my phone and then I hear the doctor say, “Daughter, Daughter! You make sure dad gets his medicine!” and when she reached for it, he turned to give it to me. She had this ugly look on her face.

My stepmother and I were talking, and she told me about the son dad had by another woman. She told me of how this woman had harassed them. The woman had called her on her job and told her to tell my dad that she was having his baby. WOW! She gets off work to tell dad about the phone call, and of course, dad denied it. The woman would ride by the house slowly whenever she sees them, then she honked the horn at them. They had a DNA test and dad was the father. After hearing this story, I wanted to find my siblings. Dad had a total of two outside kids while they were married. I was also told about the daughter. He had six children and did not acknowledge but one. I became determined to find my brother and sister.

Connecting with My Sister

My uncle Jabo came to me one day mad because my auntie was always bringing up his skeletons but keeping my dad’s secrets. He tells me that a letter had come to my aunt’s, or she found out that he was put on child support for a 9-year-old boy in Akron, Ohio. He said that they are always upholding Alfonza, but he has a little girl in Tennessee. I was so shocked; my brother had mentioned this to me once before. I remembered that when we went to visit that one of dad's friends said, "So Al, you have three girls?" I thought he was thinking that my daughter was dad's daughter too. I just ignored it. I could not wait to ask my dad. I call dad with idle talk. Then I hit him with, "Dad do you have another daughter?" He paused…Then he said, "I didn't want you guys to think less of me." I said, "Dad, you are not the first man to get a child while being married and you won't be the last one…We need to know who our sister is." He kept babbling on. He gave me a name and I tried everything I knew to find her, but I couldn't find her. Dad kept saying her mom wouldn't let him see her and her mother was crazy. I said, "Well, she might be crazy with you, but she won't be with me." I was anxious to find my sister.

Dad passed in 2015, the other two children were not listed on the obituary. In September 2018, my daughter calls me and told me that a girl messaged her on Facebook saying she was my sister. I told her that I do suppose to have a sister and to get her number for me. She texted me the number and I realized that this number had called me, and I declined the number. I thought it was a telemarketer. I went back to listen to the message. My sister, Inger, and I were so excited. I called her and when she answered I said, "Hello?" and then she said, “Hello?” There was a pause and then finally I said, “I’ve been looking for you since 1999!” She said, “I have been looking for y’all too!” We started talking and catching up. One of dad’s friends told her about dad’s passing but did not give her details of when and where was the funeral. Her husband is a Sherriff, and he had this detective to look us up after she found the obituary online. She knew so much about us. She didn’t know about the little brother who I am still looking to find but, we have been in contact ever since. I have grown a special kind of love for her and the children. My sister was 26 years old when we reached out to each other. She is one year older than my daughter.

I just hate that we didn’t meet when she was younger. She had a hard life. She said having a dad that was a married man took a toll on her life. He basically did not fight for her either. Her stepdad adopted her too. Men don’t understand how their actions affect their children. Dad expected his kids to respect him because he was our dad. It was hard to respect someone that hasn’t been there for you. She felt as though Mary did not care for her either. It was so fascinating on how much the way dad treated us the same which isn’t a good thing. I am so glad to have her in my life now.

Dad and I bonded more in eight months than we did in 48 years. We talked about everything. He overheard me talking to my daughter when she was in college. She needed $30 so when Mary came home, he told her to go get $40 out of his account to send to Jakeyla. I was surprised. I told him that I got it but he said no and that he wanted to send it to his granddaughter.

The next day my stepmother told me that if I need money to ask her and not dad. I told her that I didn't ask him for anything. When I told dad, he said that he told her that I didn't ask him for any money, and that he wanted to do this for baby girl. He also told me that he wanted to give me some money for helping him. I said that I have money coming in and he didn't have to give me any money. He went ahead and told Mary to give me $100. She waited until my brother and his wife were around and said, "Here Jackie…Your dad said you wanted some money." I told her that I didn't tell dad I needed anything. I was mad as fire. I told dad what she did, and he said I told her I was giving you that money because you were helping me. I said it was embarrassing because she made it seem like I was getting your money. I have been spending money on you and me every time we go somewhere. He said, "Yeah, I know." Honestly, I think she was afraid of us having a bond, or she didn't want me to be involved in his affairs. I wasn't trying to take over, I was trying to help, but she felt threaten. I didn't want to leave dad, but I had to go before it got ugly.

I love the time I spent with my dad in those months and he was pleasant to be around. We had a lot in common. I am so glad that we got to spend that time together. I felt at peace when he passed because of the closure. He explained a lot of things that I needed to know. When he had his last stroke, which damaged his brain, he could no longer talk. I felt helpless. I wanted to help him. When I heard the words that "It's nothing else we can do but make him comfortable." It made me numb. I could not understand that he was not going to be here for me to fallout with or call. Seeing my dad cry was hurtful. The waiting and decisions were exhausting. He would do good and then drop down. It was so stressful.

At that time, we did things as a family. My stepmom, brothers, Raman and Robert, sister, Inger, and I discussed everything that was given to us. It was hard deciding whether he would get resuscitated. Dad had talked about if he were in this situation that he did not want to be living on a machine. Inger did not want to give up on Dad. She was against it. I think because she did not get the closure that she needed.

Taking Care of My Niece

My brother had a daughter that was mixed, and we could not see her. She was on Facebook and her brother was flirting with her, so her dad intervenes and says you guys are brother and sister. She was about 13 years old when we could be around her. Her name is Audra. Audra had called me while I was at a football game. She told me that her mother had jumped on her. I was so mad. I was also one hour and a half away from her too. I called my sister to go pick her up until I got back home.

When I got home, Audra tells me that she walked in on her mom and her mom jumped her. I could not believe this was happening. Who does that? I took her in with me. We both had to adjust to each other. Audra was accustomed to a typical white girl way of living, so it was hard on her adjusting to the black way of living. I felt sorry that she witnessed her mom doing meth and her mom telling her that she wished she was never born. I told her that her mom might not have wanted you to be born but I am glad that she was born. I tried to compensate for her mom's anger and words. I would allow her to hang out with her friends. She was familiar with hanging out and coming in whenever she wanted so the rules had to be discussed, she didn't get it at first.

I allowed her to hangout with her friends, Anna and Ashley. She was supposed to be at one of her friend's house. I get a text with a picture of her hanging out at someone else's place. I was upset because she was supposed to be where I dropped her off. I did not call her, but I showed up in about 30 minutes at the house I dropped her off. Then I called her and told her that I was outside. She was panicking. At first, she told me that she went to the store. I didn't say anything. When she got in the car, I told her about the screenshot that I received. I put her on a punishment for two weeks without her phone. I told her she had from the time I picked her up until we get home to let her friends know that she will not have her phone for two weeks. She asked me was I for real and I told her yes and that you are wasting time.

We got home and I took her phone. As I am in the living room, I hear her talking. I said, "I know this girl is not talking to herself." I walked in and she was on the house phone. I said, "Audra! You are not supposed to be on your phone!" She said, "I thought you meant my cellphone." I said, "Okay since you want to be slow, let me break it down.

Don't get on anything that ends in phone. Microphone, telephone, cellphone, iPhone, or any phone that involves you talking to someone that is not in the same place as you." She started crying and said, "I can just hit my head in the wall." I replied, "Well, you better not put a whole in that wall." The punishment was two weeks without phone and don't ask to go anywhere. She had a winter dance within those weeks but for me, a punishment is a punishment. Jakeyla talked to me about letting her go. Her mom had threatened to come to the dance, and I was waiting. She did not show up.

Audra began to want to see her mom, and I did not mind if she kept her hands to herself. Her mom was cool until I asked her to send the money that Audra was getting from my brother. She then tells Audra that she wanted her to come home. My brother and I were against it. She went over to see her mom, but she wouldn't let her leave, so I called my brother and told him, and he called DHR. They went to the home and found drugs and gave her a drug test. Then they had to call the fathers of the children. Audra's mom was cursing and acting a fool. She wanted my brother to take a drug test too. He agreed to take a test but the lady from DHR said it wasn't necessary and he could take Audra home. He signed the papers and then brought her to me.

My brother went to have Audra's money sent to him so he could give it to her every month. It was a help because I was receiving disability. It was not enough for two people to live on. We started off good until Audra started to see her mom. She gradually became rebellious. She would then stay with her uncle some until she started acting up and her mom would show up unannounced trying to get her. Her mom never did this with me, so she was back with me. I explained that I would not tolerate how she acted over her uncle's house at my place. We had a meeting with DHR, it was discussed that I would have custody of her until her mom gets herself together.

Her mom would have visitations. The first visit, she was supposed to take her shopping. Audra gets to talking and reveals that they stayed at her home watching videos. I was so angry because of the lie. The next time, I only allowed her to go to visit and I would pick her up. This time, a strange man was there, and he kept getting in our conversation. I apologized to him like, "Excuse me, but who are you?" "You don't have anything to say in this matter." I was discussing getting full custody with her mother so that I could make more choices in her school and anything else. I left Audra to talk to her mom. She came to the car and told me (not ask me but tells me) that she is going to just stay with her mom.

I was on the phone with my friend Stephanie. I said, "Um no you are not! You go and tell your mom that you are going home because you don't tell me nothing." She goes in and comes back…by now I am venting to my friend Step. I said, "I'll take her to DHR and let them handle this." She comes back to the car yelling at me saying, "I don't want her to be with her mom!" I said, "You called me, and you don't yell at me!" She said something and the next thing I knew, I had grabbed her by the neck and told her girl, you don't know who you are messing with! I could hear Step saying, "Girl, you are going to jail. You know you are taking her to DHR tomorrow." I let go.

I could not believe that this chick was turning on me. I decided then that she will go back to DHR. We rode in silence down the road. I had all kinds of thought going through my head. I took this girl into my life and sacrificed for her to have the things she needed on my fixed income. I started a part time job jeopardizing my check just so we could have the necessary money. I did not care that she wanted to be with her mom, I was upset that she was talking to me disrespectfully. She did not realize I was that aunt that would knock her out. She came awfully close to being dragged. She did not like the rules that I had. She was used to hanging out, coming in late, and smoking. I found cigarettes in her jacket. I threw them away; I knew she wasn't going to ask me for them because she wasn't supposed to have them. I talked to my brother about what was going on with her. He was in agreement with me.

The office was closed until Monday; But Monday morning at 7am, I told her to get up while I packed everything she had in my vehicle. I was talking to Step again. Audra says very smartly, "You just gone take me and drop me off at DHR?" I said, "Yes!" Then she said something that ticked me off… I jumped across the bed at her. Step was yelling in the phone, "Don't you do it!" I calmed down. But I still took her to DHR. I arrived at the office to talk to the lady. I explained that I could no longer let her live with me because she is accustomed to the white way of living with time outs whereas I am used to the black way of living where we knock you out. The DHR lady kind of laughed. She said, "Mrs. Cowlin can you keep her until next Friday until the mother finds someone in the family to let her live with them?" I agreed. It was so awkward after this. I was so hurt. I had her for about 7 months. She went with her mom and starts to think that she has balls.

They were laughing, giggling, and whispering. Girl, you better ask someone about me. I cut balls off! I started thinking about what had led us to this point and I got upset all over.

We met with her mom and the DHR lady. Audra was very cocky while her mom was there. My brother showed up. He was upset too. Nobody in her mom's family wanted to deal with her. That was a sign for me. The lady came to me in private and pleaded for me to take her back until her 18th birthday. She said apparently you are the only one that can control her. "Mrs. Cowlin, you don't want anyone you love to be put in the system especially a girl… It is not a place for her." At that moment I did not care where the little heifer went. She tried to test me and I have a reputation to uphold. I told the woman no because I might hurt her. My brother said it had to be my decision because where he lived, she could not live with him. After I calmed down, I agreed to let her continue to stay. She eventually got to live with one of her mother's friends. I still supported her. Audra texted me out of the blue saying that she was glad that I entered her life. It meant a lot to me. Although we had a rough road, I loved her.

Shoes on the other Foot

I don't mind advice. I had several friends that would give me their thoughts on what they would do if it was them, but the problem was this, when it happened to them the story changed, and the end did too. I had a friend that would always tell me that she wouldn't put up with the things that my ex-husband was doing. I didn't get upset with her about her opinion. We all have them. We had lost touch, but she had gotten married and we were living in the same city.

Several years later we hooked up. I was glad to be in touch with her because she is a good friend. She came over and we began to catch up with each other's lives. I told her that my ex-husband hasn't changed, and she began with the opinions. Some weeks later she came over to the house looking like she was running for her life. I asked her what was wrong and she told me that her husband was after her. I said he better not come here with that mess around my daughter plus my ex-husband was not home. She saw her husband pulling up. I went and got my gun and came out on the porch. I told him that if he puts one toe in my yard, that they will be zipping him up in a black bag. You are not coming around here with that mess. He got back in the car and left.

I told her that I don't mind helping her, but she cannot bring this to my house. My ex-husband has never raised his voice at me in front of our daughter let alone hit me and I am not going to have anyone else come here doing that. She understood. She left and went to her parents' home; we did not talk for a while. Maybe a month later, I called to check on her. She told me that he had been begging her to come back. She said that she wasn't going back. She did.

She came to my house upset and looking like she had been fighting. She had. This time she came back to surprise him and walks into their apartment and he's in the bed with another woman. He jumps out of the bed and jumps on her. They are fighting while the other woman is still laying in the bed. He grabs an iron and draws back to hit her, and she yells to tell him that she is pregnant. He puts the iron down, grabs her and kisses her and tells her to leave for 10 minutes while he gets rid of the other woman. Now, I am stunned at what I am hearing. I said, "He asked you to leave?" ... "Wait a minute he jumps on you and he's in the bed with another woman?" I said, "You know what… Lamar has never done any of this, but if he did, girl I would be holding a number across my chest." So disrespectful. I did tell her that I would rather a man cheat on me than beat on me. She did not go back to him.

I try not to judge people's relationship because love is a strong emotion. It will make you tolerate things that you know is not good for you or good to you. It is also easy to tell someone what you would not do until you it happens to you.

Shoes On the Other foot

One of my husband's family members had the upmost respect for me. She was tired of him cheating and the disrespect of having an outside child, so she comes home and asked me if she could pay for a divorce. I was honored, but I could not let her do this because I was still in love with this man and I had faith that the marriage would work one day. I knew deep down that I was in this by myself. I explained to her that I had to decline her offer. I told her that I would be divorced on papers, but my heart would still be loyal to him. She said she would never understand it, but she loves me and that the offer was on the table whenever I was ready.

She got married some years later. I got a call from her telling me she needs to see me when she comes home. I am always glad to see her. She comes by and she apologizes to me for what she said about the divorce. She said, "Jay, I never understood what you meant when you said that you were still in love with your husband despite the things he had done until it happened to me." She went on to say, "My husband was cheating on me too. I thought I could just up and leave. I got angry and left once and then the next time I put him out, but I was still in love with the man. Then he got a woman pregnant. I thought okay this is it. But it wasn't. I still tried to be there and help him to take care of the child. But then, he wants to hit me, I then had to leave. I thought about all that I had went through with this man, then it hit me. This is what Jay was talking about." I said, until your heart is tired of hurting, you will continue to support him. When the heart is tired, then it will be time to go. Sometimes people realize too late that what they had was good.

Chapter 7

Heaven Can Wait

Every day I wake up I thank God for allowing me the opportunity to be great because I could've been dead and gone with the things that I have experienced. But because He's not ready for me yet, I'm still here. I think quite often about the things He presents to me about being patient and His plan for me. Throughout everything, I thank Him. I don't want people to cry for me because of these illnesses I've endured because it has built my character. It has strengthened my relationship with my family and God. I would have never made it if it was not for my family, friends and my God. See, my faith and my relationship with God is stronger than ever!

Today I ask you to give Him thanks for all the bad as well as the good because without the bad, you would not have known your strength. Because I was broken, I could not follow His plan… God's plan. I went through a lot to find that I had a destination that God wanted me to follow. I kept ignoring His plan for me. He continued to show me how blessed I am and that my journey was a testimony for others to hear and be inspired. I was broken down into pieces and the pieces broke down into even smaller pieces. Because I was broken, my life was a struggle. I struggled through a bad marriage, being a single parent, infidelities, lupus, and cancer.

I have lived long enough to learn that everyone is not there for or supportive of you. People of the same blood can be envious of what you have going for you. I learned that every friend is not your friend. Friends can be the most dangerous enemy that you can have. Think about it…This so-called friend has access to your life. They know all about the good, bad and the ugly. These things make those kinds of friends dangerous. It became self-evident to me at the lowest of my life what a friend is or how supportive family is.

I had broken myself down to their expectations and I was growing into a robot. I had to be strong for others, keep everyone happy, and be at their beckoning call. I became a personal assistant without pay. Although they expected things of me, they still insisted that I needed to slow down or take care of myself. I had to learn early in life that everybody is not there for you when you are down and struggling and when you need them by your side.

I am grateful that I can tell my story of how God rebuilt a broken woman and made her into a much stronger woman than she ever thought she could be! The journey that I endured was long and hard but necessary to execute God's plan. The trials and tribulations were put in motion for me to become the woman I am today. My story is the truth and it happened in my life. I would question His plan and wouldn't follow through, but He didn't give up on me. He continued to show me that I was special.

There were nights that I would pray consistently for relief of a broken heart and soul. I wanted to stop hurting. I needed to be free from this man. I was trying to keep up an image that we were okay. I wanted a father in my daughter's life. My biological father was never there for us as kids. I don't think he had acknowledged us unless we were in his presence. He signed his rights over when I was 10 or 12 years old. My dad thought that respect had to be given because he was my dad. It's not that way with me. This man was supposed to protect his little girl. I kept trying to keep hope alive. After so many attempts, lies and bumping heads, I let it go. My father was the first man to ever hurt my heart.

I stepped on pieces that seemed to cut me to the core. I often tried new approaches to avoid stepping on the broken pieces. It did not work. Instead of avoiding the pieces, I decided to pick up the pieces and use them to help strengthen my plan. When I picked up the first piece, it felt great! I put it away because it did not fit my life. This piece was my marriage. I was tired of the cheating and the back and forth with him. I was tired of being loyal to a man that didn't appreciate or deserve what I was giving unconditionally. I had to decide whether it was worth it or not. It was not a piece of the puzzle.

When I decided to put my life in perspective, it seemed to become clear. I wasn't afraid or secretive anymore about the details of my life. I did not want anyone to know about the marriage, the struggles, and the cancer. I used to be quiet about my life. I was embarrassed because of what people were saying about me and how people felt about me. I woke up from the broken pieces of my life and started putting the pieces in perspective. I was blindsided by things in my life that took a drastic toll on me. At one point I did not know if I could handle everything that came at me. I did not think that I was strong.

I did become weak when I felt like I was alone on this journey and had nobody to help me through it. I had people that I love to put knives in my back and heart. I was never the same person. It is true that sometimes an enemy can be someone you know. When I started observing my surroundings, the snakes started to appear. I have never revealed what I know to the ones that put those knives in my back and heart. Instead, I kept them out of my business.

I could never pretend to be a friend if there was some deceitful thing that transpired between me and another. Everyone thinks that I am a good woman and I think that I am, but I am human. I have anger and love too. I do not let people tell me that I must be okay with someone just because I am down or sick. Why should I? My feelings have not changed. I still don't like them, and God knows my heart. Does this make me to be a bad person because I did not want to speak to so-in-so? I think that the better person is the one who acknowledges that they are not going to be okay with a situation just because. I get that a lot. "You should be the better person." When can someone else be the better person?

I was still trying to fix me, and I was broken very badly. I was separated, dealing with lupus, raising two children, had my daughter, a niece, struggling with the bills and helping others. Whenever I told my family about what my life was like when I was married, it was when I was done. It was over. I don't get people. I continued to talk to my ex-husband, although he did not do right by me. People see that as "I still want him" or "that I am waiting on him". That is not the case. I am in a good place with myself, and I have never been insecure which makes me powerful.

I realized that for me to be blessed, I had to not be stressed. I knew that what we had took two people and one person trying to do it for two would not work. I began to listen to my God's message. He continued to show me that I was a survivor. He continued to show me how blessed I was and that He was saving me for greater things. I have two illnesses: Lupus and Cancer. One is not silent and unseen which is Lupus and the other one is seen and is known as Breast Cancer. Both can make you want to give up on your life, your dreams, your family, and friends. It became a test for me to see where loyalty lies. It weeded out who was supportive. I was incredibly surprised at the outcome. But it didn't stop me from taking care of myself.

I was strong. I used to ask questions every time my life was spared. Each time someone would come to me in a vision and say to me that God's not through with you yet, I wasn't listening. I thought that because I wasn't in church every Sunday, how could God have a plan for me. At least, there were people who made me feel that way.

My family thought I was helpless and could not help myself at times. I never knew how powerful I could be during this ordeal. Lupus had rebuilt my faith in God. I became a walking testimony, but I did not know how to tell this testimony.

As I prepared myself for the battles ahead, I had to size up the things that were in my path. I had to get informed of how to defeat my opponents. It was so many things coming at me. At first, I was scared, but I gave birth to a beautiful baby girl who made me realize that I had to be strong. Weakness could not be a part of my life. I could not be scared. I believe that I wouldn't be here if I hadn't given birth to her. I would have given up on life. She has given me so much encouragement.

When I was diagnosed with Lupus, it took me to a place that helped me to discipline myself. I didn't know much about Lupus and that made it dangerous. I took it on not realizing that it was serious. Lupus took me to a growing place with GOD.

Then when I was diagnosed with Breast Cancer, I felt the test of faith. Cancer was a test for my family and me. It helped to develop a closer relationship. I realized that my family did care about me, and they realized just how much I contributed to their lives. We needed each other.

Melissa Buckner

I had this friend from high school who was highly intelligent and would do anything to help someone especially if they were trying to better themselves. Her name was Melissa Buckner. We started hanging out and became good friends after high school. We started working at KFC during the summer and continued working while going to college. She was seeking a degree in Law, and I was seeking a degree in business. We were ambitious women.

She thought that I was a beautiful thin chic. That's what she would call me. One day we went shopping and went into this store named Lane Bryant. As I was looking around, I saw a cute shirt, but I noticed that it didn't have my size, so I yelled at the salesperson. I said, "Excuse me, do you have this in a size 8?" Melissa ran over to me and said, "No, they don't!" then she tells the salesperson, "Don't worry about her, she just playing." Melissa says, "Jackie;

they don't have anything in a size 8 with yo' thin tail. I haven't worn a size 8 since elementary. I'll take you down to the next store for thin chicks." I just laughed.

Melissa had called me to come to sit with her at her job. I didn't want to, so I made excuses as to why I couldn't come. I said that my mom wouldn't let me use the car. Melissa called back and asked my mom could I use her car to come to her job. Mom said yes...I was mad, but I went. When I get down there, we were talking about a lot of things. She told me that she wanted to be in my wedding when I married Lamar. I was confused because Lamar and I were not on good terms and I wasn't committed to anyone at that point, but she liked Lamar. She thought that he was a handsome bad boy. During the night she was talking about she didn't think she was going to graduate and had a paper to turn in the next day which was her off day. I told her that she was going to graduate.

This guy came in and she introduced us. His name was James Clark. He kept asking me questions and saying things to impress me, but it wasn't doing a thing for me. I had this weird feeling about him, and I expressed my feelings to Melissa. She said he's alright, but he wasn't alright with me. She says that he was going to help her out in closing the store by stocking the cooler. Melissa usually closes the store at 11 pm. On this night, she made me leave at 10:45pm because she knew I had to be at work at 6am the next day. I told her that I could stay. She said to me, "No chick, you got to work tomorrow." I said, "It's on 15 more minutes before you close." But she made me leave. When I walked out the door, she told me that she loved me and I told her that I love her too, chick. As I walked out the door. I felt weird. I sat in the car for a few minutes to look at her and she waved at me. A car drove up to get some gas, so I left my friend. I felt sad, but I still left. The next day was when I found out why I felt strange. Someone contacted me and said she was killed.

On May 15, 1990, I got a call that tells me that Melissa was killed at the store where she worked that morning. I told them that was impossible because she had told me the night before that she did not have to work that morning. I knew this because I had gone to her job the night before to hang out with her. We laughed and talked and saw a lot of old friends that night.

I was so confused, so I asked how many bodies they found because they only kept saying Melissa. I told them that it was someone with her last night named James. The caller said just Melissa. I called the police and told them that someone was with her. They told me to go to the crime scene and talk to the officer. I went down to the crime scene, and I see her car...I felt weak. I felt like I was going to pass out. I felt hurt. I went to the officers and told them about the guy who was helping her last night. I described him and what he had on. I told them that he had a knife, and that I had a bad feeling about him.

The officer told me that Melissa was stabbed. I thought that if I had stayed it wouldn't have happened. The guy was a drug addict. They found him in the motel with the money. The murder was also caught on camera. How could someone do this to someone that was trying to help them? I stopped believing in God and going to church. I could not understand. I cried for days. I kept trying to make sense of the situation. I remembered that she wanted me there that she called my mom. I remembered that I was mad about it. I remembered that this was her wanting to say goodbye to me. She needed for me to know that she loved me. Melissa was stabbed over 20 times by someone she knew and trusted. He got life without parole. This guy, James Kelley, killed her for drugs. He tried to steal her car, but she was the only person who could crank her car. They found him at a local hotel with the money.

Chapter 8

I Am My Sister's Keeper

February 2019

My sister, Inger, is diagnosed with Cancer. She has done well with her treatments. I prayed to God that he protects her form the things that I had endured with this disease. I did not know how strong my sister was and wanted very much to protect her from this thing. She was there for me throughout my whole ordeal, and I was going to return the favor.

When she was losing her hair, I knew just how she felt. She called me and wanted me to go with her to get her hair cut. We get there and I see that she has the patches. I knew then that it all had to go. I tell her that if she gets the bald, I would too but she had to go first. I felt like she would have backed out. She gets the cut, and she is beautiful. I kept telling her that she was because she was. Her green eyes were popping. She looked in the mirror and she's okay with it. This is what big sisters do.

Let me talk about my sister, Inger, known by many as "Popeye". She was an extraordinarily strong woman who I admire very much. When she was diagnosed with cancer, I was angry. I was afraid for her, but I thought that everything would be ok. I even told her that. I was wrong about that she would be ok. She passed; I was afraid. My sister Inger and I were remarkably close. I was unsure if I had done the best I could as a big sister. I began to question myself about whether she knew that she was my main concern. The more time we spent together the more I began to realize that I had to be strong for her. There were times when I was angry at her because I thought that she was giving up on life period. I finally realized that she was a fighter toward the end of her journey. I would make sure she was taken care of just like she took care of me. She made sure that I got everything that I needed, and I made sure that she had everything she needed too. We were two sisters fighting cancer together. It just made us closer and stronger. I went to all her appointments to help understand her treatments and diagnosis.

I got upset with the way things were going with her treatments, so I called to speak to the doctor and nurse about their lack of communication. I told them that I needed to be called back within the next day or I was going to report this to my doctor who was one of the heads of the office. Afterwards, I did not have a problem with any more communication with the entire staff. As a matter of fact, whenever I called, they made sure I was called back Asap! When she was hospitalized for the first time, I stayed with her every minute until she was released. I made sure the people treated her well. The nurses knew me from my prior hospitalization, and they made sure we had whatever we needed.

She had tumors outside her breast. The tumors were draining so she had to use bandages. I had to make sure the nurses changed them twice a day or more. Some of the nurses overlooked changing her bandages, but I did not allow that to happen. They wouldn't come to give her baths as though I was supposed to do it. I reported it to the supervisor who knew me. It never happened again. I would be told excuses by the staff to justify why they didn't bathe her. I knew a nurse there named Ian. He was one of the nurses that worked at the office of oncologists that I was seeing. I told Ian about what was going on but did not know that he was the supervisor. Ian told me that he would take care of it, and he did. Popeye said, "Girl, you know a lot of people." I said, "Yeah, I do, and they get things done." We were treated very well once they knew it was me.

Inger thought I was a trip, but she loved that I took care of her. Inger was quiet. She would just go with the flow, but I am not that person. I love my sister and my job is to protect her and to keep her out of harm's way. I tried extremely hard to keep her from pain. I moved in with her to keep an eye on her. Some nights I couldn't sleep because she would be in pain and moaning. I would have to ask her if she was okay or if she was hurting…I was praying continuously, asking God to take the pain away and to heal my sister. I wished I could transfer her pain to me. I was used to this kind of thing.

She depended on me to help her to make it through this. She would not do anything without involving me. I was honored and scared that I would make the wrong decisions for her. When the doctors gave her options on treatments, she would look at me. If they asked her if she has any questions, she would always look at me. Th doctors and nurses started just talking to me about here medical information. I did not play about the care of my sister. She would say to me that she never thought that I would be the one that would be taking care of her. I said God made this happen for me to be here for you. I am where I need to be.

People don't understand the bond that we shared. We've been friends since birth. We have never fought, but we have disagreed with each other- but never to where we would stop talking to each other for long periods of time. I love this woman with all my heart. I don't know what my life will be like without her to call and talk to everyday.

Inger used to be funny in her very own way. I loved when she would call to tell me something that was funny to her, but she is laughing the entire time and I cannot understand what she is saying but I'm laughing with her. We always called each other with all the gossip or news that we heard. I miss that. She was the quiet one. The one that would just let things go. She was mistreated by some that I wanted to hit in the throat for the way they treated her. I am my sister's keeper.

Inger was a beautiful 5 feet 4-inch light complexion woman with green eyes. When you see her, you would notice her smile and those green eyes. She never bothered anyone but would be there for you. She loved her son, Jaterius. Her heart and soul were dedicated to him. She would give her last for him. She was an extraordinary mother to him.

December 1, 2019

Trying to hold back the tears so my sister can't see that I am hurting because I cannot help her. I am sitting beside her having this weird feeling that things are not getting better. I feel bad for having these thoughts, but my stomach is weak, and my tears are stuck. I cannot let them fall. She is sleeping and I am weeping inside. She makes these sounds while she is sleeping that tells me her breathing is difficult. Popeye is quiet and sweet.

I started this journey with her because I am her big sister. She always gives me credit for that- I also tell her if the doctor doesn't tell her about something that I am familiar with. She will say, that is what my sister said. I can see in her eyes that she is scared and worried. She has never been in the hospital except when she had her son. Every day I try to hold this smile while hiding my concerns about her. I talked to God, asking him what it is you are trying to tell us. Tell me? Lord, she is a good woman. She has faith in you and so do I.

When my sister passed, I began to feel guilty. My sister was the healthy one all these years. I was the one that had been battling Lupus, and then Cancer. It seemed like it should have been me to pass. The one that everyone was prepared for. It did not seem to be fair. Why was it her? I know we are not supposed to question God's choice. I realize that she is not in pain anymore. The pain and suffering are gone. But...so was she. I will not see her again. I won't be able to talk to her on the phone or receive a text.

She would only trust to tell me of her pain. She looked up to me. I was so lost after her death because I wasn't sure that she was pleased. I tried to be strong throughout the funeral and arrangements. I wanted to make sure that everyone was taken care of at the funeral. She was gorgeous. She looked like she was sleep. I did not want to let my sister go. Although I tried months to prepare myself for this, I wasn't ready for it. We were not only sisters; we were best friends. For 50years, I had her right there for whatever...She had spoiled me during my struggles, and she made sure that my daughter and I were okay. I loved her for that.

The days that led up to her passing were hard. I felt helpless. Everyone was at the hospital to see her. Some were there that didn't visit her when she was home. I was a little upset, but mom wanted it. I was upset because she needed to know whatever they had to say before she was leaving us.

When a person passes, there are those people who show up to be recognized. I saw the hurt in so many people who would deeply miss her.

My soul was torn between what she needed and what others wanted. I felt pressured. The sad thing is that someone had buried her before she passed. I was infuriated when I received a call telling me that they were sorry for my loss. I was puzzled because my sister was still breathing and talking…I immediately told them that Popeye hasn't passed. Then I was told who had said this. I was hurt. Why would you tell that lie? I had to sit there quietly looking at them. I did not mention this to anyone.

When the doctor told me that he needed to see the family to talk about the next steps, I did not tell them until the very last moment. The doctor came in to inform us about the last days of my sister's life. My mother and sister could not bear the options that we were given. They walked out. I sat down beside my sister who was peaceful. I said, you know we got to talk about what you want. She said I know. As she searched for words I said, "You know I have Jay." She said, "Yes, take care of him." Then she said, "I want to go home." I said, "Okay." She said, "When I go, I want to be home." I was sitting there trying to hold back the tears because I had to tell my little sister that if we unplugged the machine, she would not make it home. Lord, I just ask you to help me with the words. So, I explained to her that she would not be able to go home. She looked at me and said, "Okay, I'm Okay." This was the hardest thing that I ever had to do in my life. I was so broken inside. I was hurting and I could not let my sister see this because all she has ever seen in me was strength.

The next doctor came in to confirm what the first doctor had told us, but my sister was getting weaker, and her breathing was getting low. They would have to put her on a breathing machine. I sat on the bed next to her, holding back the anger and tears because I had to tell my sister that she could not go home and that if they take the machine off, she will pass. She nodded her head that she understood.

I was broken inside, but I needed her to see strength. I saw her strength. I told her that I loved her and was proud of her. She just smiled. She said, "Mom went to make calls? I said, "Yeah." She said, "Ugh!" I giggled and hugged her. Jay, her son, didn't have time to just get this to sink in before people started to gather. I wanted family and friends to come. Just not then. Mom was on the phone contacting people. I just wanted that moment with us, her son, my mom, dad, sisters, and brother. Just us. I needed that with her. Popeye did not like a lot of attention.

Facebook Post 3/5/2020

March 5, 2020, I had to experience the loss of a sibling. My sister was my first friend. We did everything together. When she was diagnosed with Breast Cancer, I had no idea that it would lead to death so quickly. I was so scared.

I moved into her house to help my nephew. It is hard living in a place where there are so many memories of her... of us. Days after the funeral, we were going through her drawers trying to find pictures and my daughter finds a little notebook that she had written to me.

The letter went like this:

Sister not only are you fighting, I am also. I have been with you since day one and will be there until. When I see you smile it just makes my smile bigger, because I know you are a fighter, we are on the battlefield together, I will never leave your side. We will fight until victory is won. To you my sister- don't give up, never give up.

I love you!

Sister not only is you fighting
I am also. I have been
with you since day one, I
~~with~~ will be there until. When
I see you smile that just
makes my smile bigger, cause
I know that you are a
fighter. We are on the battlefield
together, I will never leave
your side, ~~I want you here
with me~~. We will fight until
Victory is won. To you my sist
don't give up, never give up.
I Love You!

Popeye left this world with a beautiful mark on my life. She was there for my daughter and me. She made being a big sister easy and fulfilling. There is not a day that goes by that I don't miss or think about her. The memories on Facebook just make me understand that we had a wonderful bond. I find myself being empty without her. I want to make her proud of me.

Being my sister's keeper became the best journey that I could have ever traveled. We already had a bond, and this Cancer thing somehow made our bond stronger with much respect between us. We were more than sisters; we were best friends. Although I miss her dearly, I am happy to know that she is not in pain anymore. She is not suffering and had peace with herself before she passed. God truly blessed me with an amazing sister, and he has given me all that I needed to be what she needed to fulfill her journey.

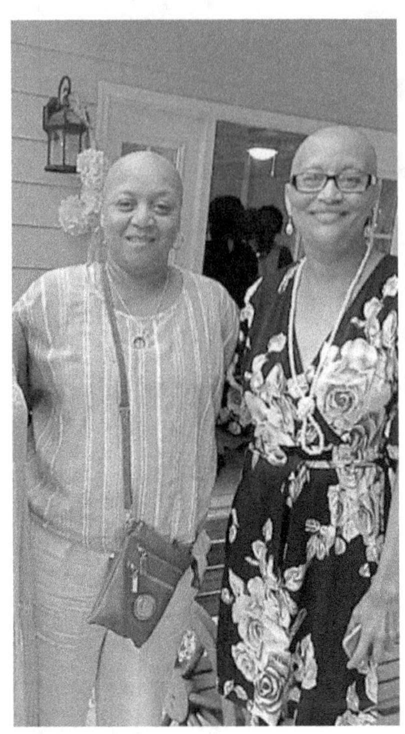

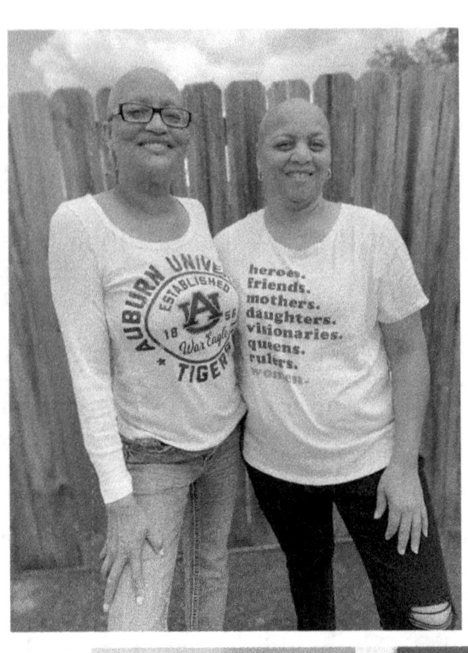
AUBURN UNIVE
ESTABLISHED
War Eagle
TIGERS
heroes.
friends.
mothers.
daughters.
visionaries.
queens.
rulers.
women.

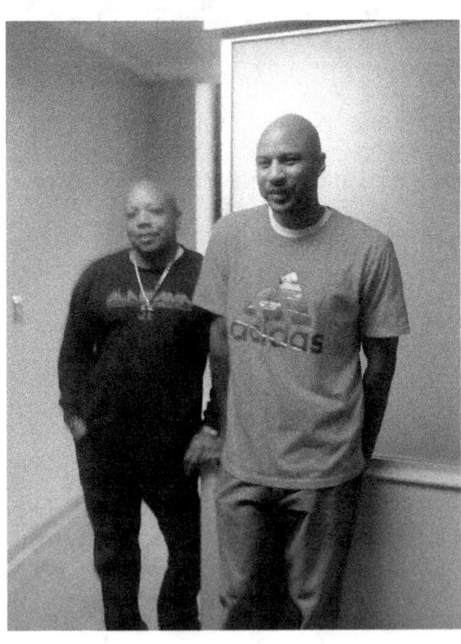
adidas

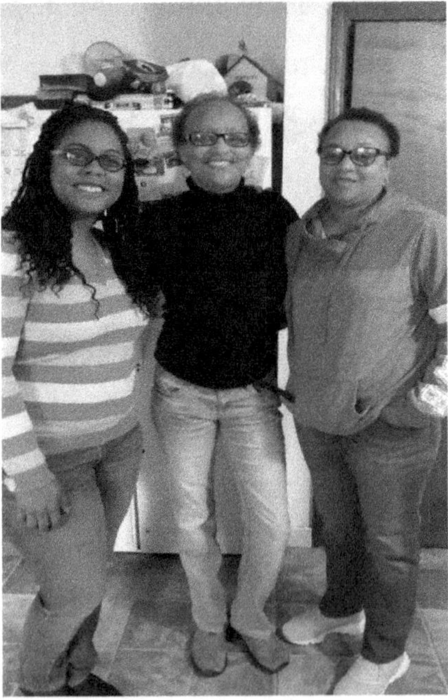

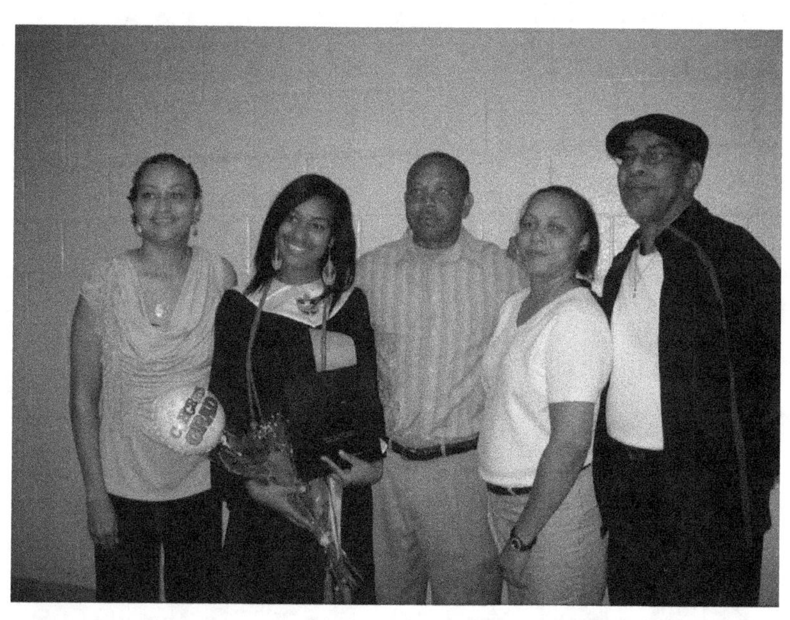

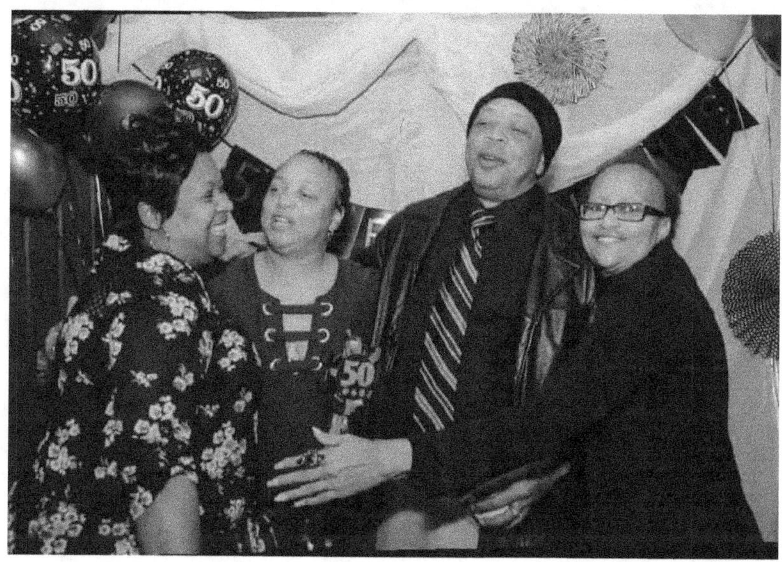
50
50
50

About the Author

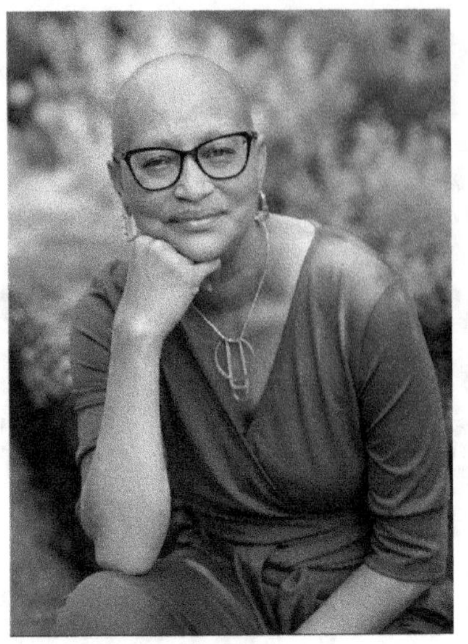

Jacqueline Regina Cowlin was born in the small town of Goodwater, AL and is strength in human form. The divorced mother of two children has one grandson and received a Master's in Business Management in 2010 at Virginia College of Birmingham, Alabama. In 1993, at the age of 26, she was diagnosed with Lupus after giving birth to her daughter. In 2017, at the age of 50, she was diagnosed with Stage 3 Breast Cancer. The two diseases and other events has given her the strength to write this book to encourage and inspire others that they are stronger than whatever they may be going through. Jacqueline is also grateful that the relationship between her and her ex-husband is good. She decided that she needed peace and realized that all that anger and hurt was taking her energy. As a result, she decided that she had to forgive him to have that peace. They are in such a better place now.

About the Publisher

Established in 2013, CoolBird Publishing House is a division of CoolBird Studios, LLC. To learn more about CoolBird Publishing House and our services, visit www.coolbirdstudios.com.

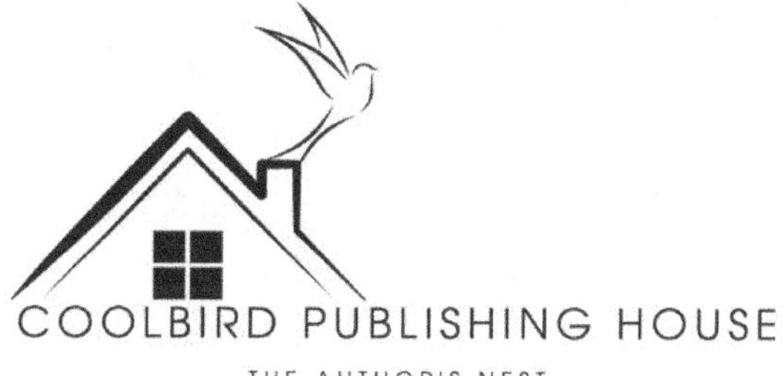

www.ingramcontent.com/pod-product-compliance
Lightning Source LLC
LaVergne TN
LVHW010105170826
845678LV00012B/2248